Spiritual Medicine

A Guide for Clinicians, Educators and Researchers

This book is dedicated to my daughter, Lisa, and to my many teachers over many years.

First Edition 2010
Second Printing

By Michael R. Basso, Ph.D., MBA,

Copyright © 2010 Michael Basso, Ph.D., MBA,

About the Author

Dr. Michael Basso has significant experience as a college level educator in psychology at Yale University and the University of Connecticut. His experience also includes being a consultant, researcher, newspaper columnist, engineer and organizational leader. Michael is the president of the CT Holistic Health Association.

As a lifelong learner and educator, Michael holds four advanced degrees and a variety of professional certifications.

Dr. Basso has a Ph.D. in professional psychology and biomedical systems, an MS in engineering science, an MBA with a focus on international executive leadership and an advanced interdisciplinary professional development diploma (PD) in pathophysiology, neural systems, and education. He also holds a BS in electrical engineering as part of his relevant undergraduate education. Michael is also certified in a variety of quality systems and health related areas.

Michael has made a rigorous study of religion, metaphysics and philosophy, and has published several related articles for the *Yale Journal for the Humanities in Medicine*.

Michael Basso has also published several articles in the area of clinical neuroscience.

Preface

I, Michael, procrastinated about writing my books for ages, until one day I got a wake up call that came out of the blue. The ambulance and fire truck arrived early on a Saturday morning at my neighbor's house. Next came the police. When we didn't see anybody being put on the stretcher, the situation was becoming clear.

Then came a priest, followed by a mini van driven by two gentlemen with black suits. They sat in the driveway for hours. Seeing my relatively young, fit, active and perpetually smiling neighbor being carried out in a body bag was a reminder to all about how fragile life can be and the importance of time. Seeing his elderly mom walk out of the house that day really drove the concept of applied spirituality home. As her *hope* turned to *despair*, it was clear that both concepts are part of the same continuum and that energy medicine is only part of the *spiritual healing system*.

I was once at a seminar at the Mayo Clinic and had the opportunity to ask some leaders what they thought the medicine of the future might be about. The reply was interesting to say the least. These leaders suggested that it would be more like the medicine on Star Trek*: light, sound, electro-magnetic fields, robotics,* and other forms of high tech yet to be invented. This experience and others have made it clear that it may not even be necessary to see, touch, or be near a patient to facilitate healing, even in conventional medicine. Distance healing is considered a real possibility by many credible scientists today; as is has been for eons in many traditional cultures.

Ideas about healing through photographs and the concept of the 'healing channel,' on TV, are not as far fetched as they may have been before the invention *fMRI* and a deeper understanding of the quantum world have emerged. The real thing - of course.

How did Jesus heal anyway? Was it him doing the healing or 'his dad' - or what some may call the father/mother/it called God? Or was it Jesus and God working in harmony?

Note that this little book it meant to be used as a stand alone guide or as a companion to the book - *The 13th Step: The secret of becoming a co worker with the higher power of God*

Prologue

While the *human energy field* has been considered to be an integral part of human healing for eons of time, the relationship between the energy system and human emotion are now being viewed from a teleological, or goal driven, perspective.

As the goals of emotions and thought are both becoming clearer and the underlying neurobiology and physiology are becoming more understandable, the intrinsic and extrinsic motivational drivers of human survival and existence are paving the way for the emergence of the true holistic model of human existence.

The true healing system may rightfully be considered to be that of a bio/psycho/social one, which is constrained by *culture*, influenced by *technological innovation*, and regulated by a *higher spiritual power* that is within and outside of us.

In some cultures, the source of neurological and psychological troubles may very well believed to be the result of the doings of members of a very well defined and broad *demonic hierarchy*; the antithesis of the angelic one. In other, more scientific, 'cultures,' the root of some of these problems are believed to be most likely caused by problems associated with *NMDA regulated glutamate channels* leading to *epileptiform* activity within the medial temporal lobe of the brain. Still other 'subcultures' may entertain the idea that the glutamate channels are regulated in part by zinc and magnesium and that these nutrients are in turn regulated by other nutrients, including the B Complex and that Vitamin C and Omega three fatty acids must be in balance along with a host of other factors.

The purpose of human love will be explored within the domains of survival on the one hand and divine love within a broader, more universal, context.

The truth of the matter is that it is truth that *matters most*, and authority which does not espouse truth, wherever it may be found, *matters least*. So if you find an idea or a reference that you don't resonate with, consider that the person who wrote the material, regardless of their credentials, may be at least as smart as you are in some way and that you may learn something useful that you overlooked; if even just a small amount. Might want to jot some things like that down.

A couple of pages have been added at the end so that you make notes from this book or from whatever sources suite your purposes.

Throughout this text we will discuss a variety of disease processes, including what might aptly be called the *spiritual diseases*. These are the diseases that make sufferers appear as though they have had taken away their *spirit, like they don't have a soul.*

Or more appropriately:

The soul doesn't have an effective body and mind to work through properly

This category includes those disease processes that affect our ability to connect our higher cognitive brain functions with our innate spiritual essence. This grouping would include, but not be limited to:

1) Addictions

2) Alzheimer's Disease

3) Antisocial Personality

4) Anxiety

5) Borderline Personality

6) Depression

7) Epilepsy

8) Schizophrenia

9) And so forth

Note that a brief list of 'spiritual alignment goals,' from the companion book - *The 13th Step: The Secret of Becoming a Coworker with the higher power of God*, has been included in Appendix I.

Over the years, I have noted some things that have lead to success and shut the door to errors in many areas. This list contains some of them in a hopefully catchy list that is easy to read, remember, and understand. Feel free to modify this list and to create your own as you see fit.

This gist of the list is that God tends to help those who try to help themselves and that once we make the effort to take responsibility for our lives; we tend to find an inner strength to accomplish or goals. When we are successful, our sense of self esteem grows and our confidence in our abilities grows in leaps and bounds and manifests in accomplishments.

We are aligning our *lower selves* with the *lower aspects of a higher power* that is greater than ourselves, and that may be called upon when are at our limits of self effort, and that will stop any potential dark force, real or imagined, in its tracks.

Once we are on track we are in a better position to help others and may indeed be asked to do so, without being taken advantage of.

The reader will find that through didactic materials, anecdotes and even some conjecture, that:

- They will enhance their ability to help themselves or others to study, or to teach about *spiritual concerns* by better understanding clinical diversity from a systems perspective.
- Through enhanced understanding, they will seek to find continuously improving ways to responsibly allow patients the *respect, tolerance* and *freedom* to be *co-creators and even teachers* in the therapeutic process.
- Through the deeper *understanding* gathered and the enhanced *self-esteem* gained, the more *confident* client will naturally be in a better position to be healed, and even self healed, once the blocks to enhanced self-esteem are removed piece by piece.
- While the *spiritual empowerment* process is facilitated through living philosophy, religion, metaphysics and common sense, aspects of the natural sciences, including medicine, psychology, neuroscience, and stress leadership, are seamlessly integrated into a powerful gestalt, which I like to call *Spiritual Medicine*.

- Some thoughts about some very practical clinical ideas, like ways to free a patient's spiritual essence through *nutrition, fitness, laughter, fun, programmed dreaming, counseling* and even *distance healing,* are explored.
- Spiritual medicine also includes ideas concerning ways to align the being of the patient with spiritual domains of *art, architecture* and *music* on the one hand and *ethical* social/*societal* concerns on the other.
- Provocative topics, including *divine love* and *death, dying* and *traumatic grief,* are explored head on through scientific explanation, as well as indirectly through anecdotal evidence and sensible conjecture.
- The spiritually inclined researcher will be more apt to explore evidence based, as well as anecdotal ideas, from *reductionist* as well as *holistic* views.

Please note that while the title includes reference for clinicians, researchers, and educators, that this book was also created with the student and interested layperson in mind.

Spiritual Medicine: A Guide for Clinicians, Researchers and Educators

Contents Page One

4. Preface

6. Prologue

15. Introduction

21. Teleological Perspectives on Human Existence

33. The Philosophy of Philosophy

42. Theological Views on Spiritual Healing

56. The Neurobiology of the Soul

63. Laughter, Humor, and Fun

68. Fairy Tales and Mirror Neurons

76. Dreams and Dreaming

83. Energy Medicine

94. Death, Dying, Bereavement and Traumatic Grief

108. Anxiety and Depression

115. Hope, Despair & Learned Helplessness

Contents Page Two

120. The Dark Force

133. Stress and Chronic Disease

141. Nutrition, Fitness and Spiritual Wellbeing

146. Art and Health

150. Architecture and Sacred Spaces

156. Light and Health

162. Music and the Human Nervous System

166. Ethics and Spirituality

172. The Physician of the Future

181. The Spiritual Organization of the Future

188. Divine Love

196. Pastoral Counseling

202. Epilogue

Contents Page Three

207. Notes by You and for You

209. Appendix I

Thirteen Step Program for Spiritual Wellbeing

213. Appendix II

Abbreviated Experimental Protocol for suggested studies on Traumatic Grief

220. References and Suggested Readings

241. Insights

Introduction

During the period when I was a quality and reliability engineer at a fortune 500 company, I was exposed to a variety of *energy medicine* systems and participated in lots of related courses, seminars and workshops. As an *evidenced based* statistics expert, while I was quite interested in the field, I was very skeptical about lots of claims and had expected to debunk much of what I was exposed to. To my utter amazement, the skepticism was most often proven otherwise, many times over, and in the most powerful and thought provoking ways.

In once instance, I, along with an engineer from another fortune 500 company, happened to take an energy healing course together.

Not only were we bewildered at what we saw, we were actual participants in this *very strange* world. At least it seemed that way at first.

In one case, an older woman, who was a fellow student, was not able to rotate her shoulder freely form more than 30 years. After a group of students worked on her energy field, '*Without touching her'* in any way, she went into a very deep trance like state for almost 20 minutes.

While in this altered condition, she muttered something about being in a marketplace long ago and having a robber stick a knife in her shoulder. She shrieked a bit, then jumped up and rotated her arm like nothing was ever wrong with it. Hadda be there, but she tried everything imaginable over the years with no success at all and was about to give up.

While there are a variety of views on what really happened; such as a genetic memory being erased, a past life time reprocessing, or a metaphor that she was 'making up at some level,' the absolute reality was that her arm was really free and we did not touch her *at all*.

In another case, I was attending a Ph.D. seminar in psychology, when, for the fun of it after class one night, someone applied healing energy to the field around my wrist.

During the experience, I felt like I too was experiencing several events from 'the distant past,' somehow.

The next morning, there was a short red line on my wrist that looked like a knife cut. The red mark lasted for about a month and then formed a small scar that is still visible in his wrist almost 20 years later. Once again, no one physically touched my wrist.

In more recent times, I had the privilege of witnessing an experiment at the University of Connecticut medical school in which *healing energy* had been applied to human bone cell cultures. In one dish, the cells were healthy *osteoblasts* and the other dish contained human bone cancer cells, called *osteosarcoma*.

When healing energy was applied to the healthy cells, there was evidence that the cells were thriving in *statistically significant* and *measurable* ways. The cancer cells began to die simultaneously. Again, no one touched the cells.

Many anecdotal experiences have also occurred in which both mental and/or physical conditions have been 'healed' at long distances; in some cases many miles away and in some instances without the person even knowing about the healing; the ethical issues notwithstanding.

In one case, a relative was about to undergo a biopsy for suspected metatastic liver cancer, that appeared objectively on a CAT scan.

The night before the surgery, a women who I had never met before told me that my relative "had been given another chance and that I would know what she meant the next day."

The next day I spoke with the surgeon who was flabbergasted. He said that the biopsy was negative, so he decided to perform a laproscopic analysis of the liver, through a small tube placed through the abdominal wall; again nothing was found. The procedure was then followed by opening the abdomen and *palpating* the liver. Nothing was found at all, no one touched him and the healing was done at a distance of several miles.

The relative got real cocky and promptly returned to his bad health habits, so the case also brought to mind some *ethical issues* and thoughts about karma, healing others without explicit permission, etc.

I also recall as story of a person who had dental problems with no apparent and logical reasons. He would also have a recurrent dream about being in a past war and knocking out someone's teeth with the butt of a rifle. When, coincidentally, a very intuitive person told this person that that was the reason for the dental issues, got that person thinking.

I have also witnessed several cases in which an *intuitive person* would accurately diagnose a disease in another person from a distance of many thousands of miles in some cases.

A variety of ethical issues also came to the fore during this era of exploration. Some of these observations and considerations also made clear several benefits about distance healing; besides the fact that it can really work.

Goal driven, teleological survival mechanisms, were also very apparent

Common Meditation Mantras

HU

HOO

Ra Ma Da Sa Sa Say So Hung

Om Mani Padme Hum

Om Nama Shivia

Om

Aum

Amen

One

Teleological Perspectives on Life

All living things are driven by two main goals that have been described in many ways and in many cultures through eons of time, a plethora of scriptures, and through just plain observation and common sense. Strive to survive as a physical being or strive to die so that higher goals, perhaps those that may be called *spiritual*, may be accomplished in another form – or with no form at all. Goals may also be called *teleological* drives.

A teleological perspective on living systems means plain and simply that there is a goal or are goals that may be *explicitly* in place or *implicitly* implied from an unconscious perspective. In reality, there are many interconnected goals in the complex world that we live in; some of which are mutually supportive and others which may be in conflict with each other.

In the chapter on stress, it may become clear how and why these conflicts may lead to excessive maladaptive stress and associated mental, emotional and physical illness. In this chapter, a general overview on stress will be provided.

An example of an explicit goal are the forces that help healthy baby squirrels to *survive* and which make mother squirrels want to help their babies thrive and to grow into healthy capable adults.

At another level of teleology, nature may put forces in place to facilitate the quick demise of a squirrel that was born with a serious defect. In the human condition, the same forces may be at work at a variety of different levels.

For example, at one point in an illness, the patient may want very much to do whatever it may take to overcome death and to live on.

At a later point in the life of the patient, the person may have the goal to survive as a *spiritual being*, which could perhaps include a sub goal to die a speedy death as a physical being and another goal to live on in another physical form or survive as a spiritual being in *another level of existence*, in what one may call a *spiritual world or heaven*.

The family of the patient, who really wants to be freed from their earthly chains, may have yet another goal driven perspective on the matter at hand. They may want their mom or dad, who once had a lot to do with their survival, to *live forever*, so that at some level the family members may perceive that they have a better chance of survival, even if they may lose their life savings, by forcing the patient to live on, who may want to *move on, in opposition to the goals of the family*.

This very complicated state of affairs on planet Earth has some very deep and distant roots into our *genetic past*.

Flowers, trees, and even so-called weeds have the built in goal to survive. This innate force driving us to this survival state is so strong that it may cause the plant in question to *spend its precious resources* on 'crazy stuff' like creating thousands of seed pods to assure that genetic material is passed on, or to develop thousands of leaves to capture enough sunlight to thrive regardless of future weather conditions.

Now, we humans have been around this planet for a long long time. We have been the predator and the prey and our symbiotic relationships with the plants on our planet are absolutely necessary for our survival goals to be realized.

The cues associated with survival are so hardwired into our nervous systems that even viewing a painting of the African savanna has been said to decrease a hypertensive state in some patients. Why so?

Well, the trees are readily climbable, so they can be a place to hide while in search for prey or edible vegetation in the open countryside on one hand, and/or to hide from becoming a meal on the other.

We can readily see that the survival goals of the trees are in alignment with the goals for human survival.

The survival goal for the hungry lion or shark, with an interest in a human meal, may be quite another story at yet another level or domain of survival which is in opposition to that of human survival.

The survival cues that may help us to avoid swimming in waters where dangerous sharks may be present are just as real as the tree cues from Africa, but for different *teleological reasons*.

Since our genetic (and/or spiritual) ancestors have *been food for others in the past*, there is something built into us that may automatically be getting us to prepare to *fight or flee* at the mere site of a dorsal fin on the other side of the next big wave, or on the movie screen for that matter.

While there is some dispute about the topic, and much of our reactive behavior is indeed learned, humans tend to respond more to things that are logical dangers from the past, like dangerous animals, than they are man made dangers from more modern times.

Unless of course, when someone becomes the victim of a *modern* traumatic experience, such as from a war injury or that experienced during a car accident.

Someone who has been shot from a helicopter may shudder at the sound of a safe traffic chopper flying over head.

In this case, their goal to survive facilitates another goal within their nervous systems; the development of *neural circuits* that 'tell' the organism that danger is near (real or imagined) and that in order to best survive that we must pay close attention when the traffic copters fly overhead, or we *could die*.

One of the symptoms of post traumatic stress disorder, is *hyper vigilance*; an uncomfortable state of over arousal and constantly paying attention to potential danger.

Thankfully, nature has also built in mechanisms that may help the organism to *habituate* or to eventually get used to the helicopters flying overhead. Sometimes the patient may have to re experience and process the memory of the war trauma before habituation can occur.

The human nervous system is also run *rather expensively* on glucose; which needs oxygen and a variety of other nutrients, such as the B Vitamins and certain minerals, to be metabolized.

Therefore, the goals of the *digestive, circulatory* and *respiratory* systems also need to be realized to give the nervous system enough energy to process the traumatic memories.

In order to keep the goals of an expensive nervous system intact, nature provides mechanisms to facilitate learning such as language acquisition at specific times, called *critical periods of development.*

During those periods of enhanced synaptic inter connecting, called *synaptagenesis (*making synaptic connections*)*, the goals of survival are realized in *Boolean logical functions*, including the basic AND, OR and NOT functions, which program the nervous system for optimum survival.

The goals related to *reliability* of the human system are also enhanced by a series of 'techniques' that may also be found in human industrial designs. *Redundancy* can be readily noticed in beings who may have two eyes, two lungs and two ears; while *derating* - having more than you need - can be implied within subsystems that are *adaptive* in nature. In these cases, there are reserves in place, like extra fat or glucose, just in case.

Divergent logic may be found in important structures, including the mammalian retina. These logical systems help to assure that nothing is missed, while *convergent* systems are in place to improve the signal to noise ratio of real images to garbage.

Going beyond the biological and psychological domains, the *social goal seeking* processes within the human system are also readily apparent and will now be considered from a clinical perspective.

While the goal of the healer may be to do something to someone, like heal them, whether they want to be healed or not, the goal of the patient may be to *heal themselves*, to *ask god* to heal them or to even unconsciously *go through a trying experience* on purpose to learn something important. Well, how and why Jesus died by crucifixion is something to ponder as well.

Patients may have goals that purposefully exclude attendees, including medical sales people, in terms of gender, age, methodologies or even style. The patient has the right to exclude anyone they may want to, including residents, students, observers or even their own family. Also within the social arena, patients have the right to include family members *as they see fit*.

When the *spiritual goals* of the patient are in opposition with the *power and efficiency goals* of the clinician, serious problems can result.

I once knew a woman who had a child with a serious liver disease that could have been helped significantly by the use of protein types that are readily found in chicken eggs.

This woman's spiritual goals precluded her and her child from ingesting anything made from egg products. This goal was so strong that she <u>let her child die</u> rather than have her ingest egg products.

Had her goal been to convey the message to her physician in a timely manner, and her/his goal have been to listen carefully, they may have come to a *mutually agreeable solution* in the form of a suitable vegetarian protein source which may have possibly saved the child's life.

The survival goals of the patient and her family were more in alignment with survival beyond the physical plane than within these worlds of *matter, energy, time and space* (47).

There are some religious ideas that are focused on healing associated with the material worlds and others that are more in alignment with what many religious and mystical systems call the *higher planes of existence* (105, 98, 99).

While there may be variation among the various details, the general idea is that there are what is commonly called the *astral plane*, which is supposedly like the physical plane, but comprised of more subtle matter.

Beyond, or perhaps within the astral plane is what many believe to be the *causal plane* (88) of existence. This realm of existence is believed to be where information from past deeds, called *karma* in eastern lingo, is stored. In fact, many patients believe that their current illnesses may in some way be associated with something that they did in the past, even before this lifetime, in many cases.

I once knew of a gentleman who had issues with his teeth that were unexplainable in terms of any physical of psychological causes. Shortly before serendipitously meeting and then chatting with a *medical intuitive* on the matter, this man had had several dreams in which he remembered being a soldier and knocking out the teeth of an enemy soldier with the butt of his rifle.

Astonishingly, the intuitive told this man a similar story and that this was the reason for his dental problems in this life.

While many believe that the goal of karma is to teach us lessons, others believe that much more complex processes are in place that are related to past and current life traumatic memories associated with: *what we have done to others*, *what others have done to us*, *what we have done to ourselves*, and *what we have observed others doing to others* (45).

These processes, while supposedly connected to the causal body are associated with the yet more subtle bodies of the deeper mental planes, included the unconscious mind.

Some believe that dreams and goal driven processes associated with relieving the effects of these past traumas are required to alleviate the associated illnesses that have manifested in present time.

At even more subtle and deeper levels, many religious tenets suggest that beyond these bio/psycho/social planes of matter, energy, space and time, that there are regions comprised of various gradations of *pure spirit* that humans also exist simultaneously on. (99,100,105,106)

While some religions suggest that it is the goal of human life to strive to reach these higher *heavens,* others believe that it is more important to bring spirit down to the material world, while yet others believe that it is the birthright of all humans to excel in *both major divisions of existence, the material planes and the spiritual planes* (51).

In any event, prayer, contemplation and meditation have been used extensively over eons of time to help humans balance themselves in this world. Some also believe that meditation is the key to consciously entering the more subtle spiritual planes which are said to consist of pure light and sounds, including what many religions consider to be the *word of god* (98, 51).

Regardless of the associated belief system, the right type of meditation for the right person can help one to relax (117) as manifested in changes in *brain wave frequency, skin conductance and heart rate.*

Of course, in some types of mental illness and depression, some brain regions are already oscillating too slowly, and may not adapt well to meditation. In these cases, specific types of neurofeedback, visualization, and/or music entrainment may be useful to 'speed up or slow down' one side of the cortex to achieve balance prior to commencing a meditation practice.

In any case, many believe that the meditative process is a natural one that is akin to a cat or rabbit purring with the built in *goal* of achieving balance, and that balance may also be achieve through the meditation itself.

The following exercise may be useful to the patient, clinician, researcher or educator alike and is easy to do, is done by oneself and can be very effective.

1) First choose one of the meditation mantras on page 18 of this book
2) Take *ones own* pulse for one minute and record that number
3) Sit in a comfortable position, with back straight and feet on the ground or in a lotus position
4) Take a few deep breaths and close ones eyes
5) Gently repeat the *mantra* to oneself for about 5 minutes, gradually increasing the time to 20 minutes over several weeks

6) Gently open the eyes and retake pulse and compare change in heart rate
7) The pulse taking part of this exercise is optional and may be used initially and occasionally to get an idea about changes associated with meditation
8) Note that it is important to gently ignore any intrusive thoughts or other distractions that may arise during meditation
9) Gently observing that breathing may be helpful to help one stay focused on the mantra
10) Note that some folks may prefer a longer mantra because paying attention to the mantra helps them to not pay attention to distractions

A side benefit for doing something for one self is the shift of *responsibility back to oneself*. Once successful, the associated increase in *self-esteem* for helping oneself will also increase *self-efficacy* (6), or the perception that we can be *productive* and *successful*.

Since successfully completing ones goals breed's future successes, those who take responsibility for their lives tend to be successful at being in balance, which in turn helps bring on more successes, and so on.

The Philosophy of Philosophy

When patients are seriously ill over long periods of time, it is not uncommon to find them desperately trying to learn from religion, philosophy, and many forms of what one might call, *spirituality*. The spiritual provider can not even come close to understanding their patient's purview unless they understand their personal philosophy. In this section, I have included an integrated synopsis on philosophical concepts that may be related to health and wellness.

It is recommended that not only the hospital chapel, but the spiritual practitioner's study areas also include a broad array of reading materials in religion, philosophy and metaphysics.

I agree with some broad thinkers that there is a *golden thread* running through the whole of philosophy which is a roadmap towards optimal human survival and health.

Some say that the primary goal of evolution is to spread successful genetic material far and wide. The most robust 'genotypes' would then presumably have the greatest chance of producing successful 'phenotypes,' given the constraints and limitations of the environment. Nature and nurture could then be considered as allies in the game of evolution and survival.

As each biological system struggles towards optimal and enduring survival, other systems may be competitors, while still others form symbiotic relationships. As biological systems developed in more complex environments, more complicated *strategic alliances* began to emerge on the survival front. For example, the common crow may use a complicated array of communication techniques to simultaneously secure food and safety. Survival of the individual and the successful group are testimony to the spread of stronger genes. At a variety of levels, some conscious and some not, new and important survival techniques would evolve over time. An appreciation for beauty, love, and eventually wisdom, would emerge as powerful techniques to assure optimal survival and genetic evolution.

Through untold eons of time, human systems developed complex emotions and cognitive processes to help win this struggle of life over death. As new cultures emerged, the notion of survival took on a variety of different approaches. Survival for family and working groups, plants and animals, and eventually an appreciation for tools and shelters became paramount. As more time passed, *survival through the gates of death* itself became the ultimate strategic goal for many.

Seers and mystics of various and sundry types would eventually emerge. These special individuals would communicate their ideas in every language and from many perspectives. Among the early outputs of these survival systems were included the ancient *Vedas and Upanishads*. Some say that there were much earlier tomes on survival.

The common task, from the subatomic particle to the zebra, and throughout humanity, appears to be *survive, survive, and then survive some more*. Even the drives towards the creation of art, music, dance, and verse, could be boiled down to this common denominator by the clever thinker.

As our cognitive machinery proceeded to become more refined, philosophy rose among the greatest of the healing arts in a way. From the early dawn of civilization, natural philosophers would not only develop complex strategic plans, but also detailed tactics, to insure optimal survival. From the East, systems of fitness and health were inextricable linked with divine and metaphysical overtones. Systems of yoga, Ayurveda, Chinese medicine, and a variety of related systems would eventually emerge among many other related systems.

I think that the theme of health and survival may also be seen throughout the evolution of Western philosophy. In many ways, the true philosopher is the *soul of medicine*.

At a variety of levels, humans have evolved a collective consciousness. Within this scheme there are those who tend to resonate with certain aspects of survival and others that resonate with other parts of the whole. However, the whole of philosophy may be considered to be the global view, complete with universal truths mixed of course with its share of untruth and conjecture. I see the individual philosopher as a facet reflecting part of the whole. However, none except the true eclectic philosopher would be capable of representing the whole system of philosophy and only the complete picture could reflect the optimal survival strategy.

To illustrate my point, I see the 'philosophy of philosophy' as an idyllic archetypical thread that links the best of philosophy with a universal theme: survival. Using the *Hegelian dialectic* (28) as a model for the evolution of the 'philosophy of philosophy,' each universal truth might be considered as a 'thesis' in itself. As a new facet gets added to this grand scheme, the new construct might be perceived as supporting or as being the 'antithesis' of the original construct. However, true universal constructs would add to the synthesis of the whole of philosophy. Innate drivers that mold every form, as Aristotle postulated, would of course be among the teleological factors goading survival intrinsically. The *Kantian* (28) view of solving scientific problems by combining rational thought and empirical observation would certainly have its place in this idyllic scheme.

For example, I think that the *Nicheian* (28) concept of the 'superman,' while debatable in its details might in ways reflect parts of a universal prototype for optimal individual survival. At yet another level, *'The Republic' of Plato* (28), while being perhaps full of its own dross, can be viewed as a reflection of a higher level archetype. This time the archetype is reflective of a group of groups, each one potentially reflecting a unique facet as part of an optimal survival strategy for group collaboration and cooperation.

When viewed as a composite whole, the 'golden thread through *all* of philosophy' takes on a very special meaning. Paramount within the meaningful aspects of the whole philosophical system may be seen as a puzzle with a very important goal strewn amidst its pieces. To ensure optimal survival is to ensure 'optimal health.'

From this proposed vantage point, I think that the 'golden thread through philosophy' may be seen as the *ultimate health and wellness model*. Of course, the ongoing realization of this lofty model would only be accurate if it reflected the all of philosophy that *ever was or ever could be*.

I think that the outward manifestation of the ultimate health and wellness model would then be reflected in archetypical beauty at a variety of levels and planes. Within this idyllic schema many universal philosophical constructs might be seen as drivers towards the compendium of axiomatic universal truths. The moral views of *Francis Bacon* (28), the importance of strength as noted by Nietzsche, the empirical thinking of *Aristotle* and the introspection of later philosophers are all examples of these universal drivers.

Thus, the 'universal axiomatic truths' as plucked throughout the whole tree of philosophy, including before the Vedas, might be seen as a roadmap. This roadmap, if viewed in its entirety (including links to all of science and religion), would ideally be a *preventive systems model* leading to optimal survival as reflected in optimal health. Not just optimally healthy individuals, but optimally healthy groups, and systems of groups. Of course, *the focal place of human disease, the workplace*, would eventually take on its true level of significance in preventive medicine as the philosophy of philosophy manifests.

Now, given the utopian realization of the philosophy of philosophy, what might be the role of ultimate physician? I think the role of doctor would then take on its true original meaning as teacher.

It is interesting to me that the father of medicine, *Hippocrates*, was not only a physician, but a philosopher as well. Like *Descartes*, Hippocrates was also a dualist (28). He believed that the soul ran the body, but was also a separate entity in itself. Would the archetypical physician also have a spiritual inclination, as well as being a teacher? If so, then the ideal physician could help to assure higher standards throughout the sum total of minds, or a manifestation of God in *Spinoza's* purview (28). Would the natural evolution of the 'philosophy of philosophy' be the manifestation of optimum *survival, health, and beauty* throughout the 'higher planes of existence throughout eternity', as untold philosophers have postulated?

If so, then would the genetic systems eventually 'reset' themselves towards optimal health after generations of living the 'philosophy of philosophy' manifest? Of course, nutrition, stress management, and fitness protocols would have been optimized is this utopian paradise. And what of the physician/teacher? Would the new focus be upon agronomy, architecture, art, music, nutrition, balanced exercise systems, and stress leadership? Would it also require a significant knowledge of emergency medicine, just in case? And even then would the art and science of emergency medicine being practiced within the strictest of *cultural and ethical guidelines*?

I think that the practical manifestation of the 'philosophy of philosophy' would be deeply rooted in aesthetics and demonstrated in myriad forms of *beauty*: beauty of body/mind/spirit within the context of social systems, living spaces, and multicultural diversity. Kabalistic philosophers would certainly agree. Perhaps the most important yardstick to measure success by might be called a *universal aesthetic template*. Beauty would be the outcome of 'golden thread through philosophy' manifest over long periods of time.

Of course, humanity has a very long way to go before the manifestation of 'the philosophy of philosophy' could even remotely become a living reality, if indeed it was meant to be. However, we as human systems have a very unique tool: our imaginations. That tool is constantly changing medicine, the arts, and the humanities. *Schopenhauer* (28) reminds us that the intellect tires but the will works even in sleep. I think the will towards survival is the driver of the imagination. Imagine well, my fellow humanists!

Keep in mind that patients and research subjects are in hospital settings for one of two reasons; to survive and live or to die. In accordance with these innate drives, they will resonate with people, places and things that will help them to *fulfill their goals,* one way or another.

Those with self destructive tendencies may find lots of ways to get attention, have people help them to hurt themselves, or to even try hard to die.

Even the most serious of accidents may not be an accident at all! Please do not underestimate the power of self destruction and *fear of abandonment.*

It is also important to consider that belief has lots to do with someone's actions, whether they may be conscious of unconscious in nature.

For instance, those who believe in an afterlife, or another life for that matter, may have very different solutions to their perceived roles as a physical being and/or a spiritual being.

Much of Theology evolved out of philosophical ideas.

~Does the Body have a Soul or does the Soul have a Body or Both? ~

Theological Views on Spiritual Healing

To really understand your study subjects, clients or students, it is important to communicate clearly with them about things that are important to them. To reach an understanding about where they may be spiritually, it is very important to reach a state of reality with them by knowing materials that are pertinent to their spiritual backgrounds.

A side benefit of knowing the religious systems that they resonate with would also be a better understanding about their *levels of hope, their views on an afterlife,* and *their levels of tolerance* and *special requirements.*

For instance, a person who is planning a special way to pray several times per day may be best rooming with a hospital mate that is tolerant and accommodating. And please assume that the requirements of devote followers are *not negotiable.*

By having a broad background regarding common and uncommon religious systems, the *spiritual advisor* will be better able to predict relevant *stressors* and pertinent *behavior patterns.*

Having gained an understanding about a variety of religious systems, a better view on common themes and differences, the spiritually trained clinician will also have the opportunity to gain greater tolerance of those with differing belief systems.

A sick and highly stressed person will readily pick up on those who are in disagreement with them, especially when it comes to the things they may be ready to even die for; their religious convictions.

When I was a kid growing up in Connecticut and New York State, it was common to hear of a few faiths, including Catholic, Protestant Sects, Jewish, Baptist, and occasionally Islam. As I got older, religions, including, Buddhism, Hinduism, Wicca, Christian Science, Radhasoami, Scientology, and even Satanism with its many sects, were becoming popular in the media and among people that I knew and hung out with sometimes. Even TV shows about Pentecostal snake religions began to emerge in the media.

Mystical/philosophical groups including Astara, Theosophy, The Rosicrucians, Freemasonry, and Self-Realization Fellowship are among the many that have become popular, albeit often controversial, in the United States alone.

Popular books, including *The Secret Teachings of All Ages* (40) by Manley Hall, have shaken the roots of nearly all conventional, and perhaps many not so popular, religions that your patients have once believed wholeheartedly in. The *hospital chaplain* or the *pastoral counselor* unaware of such 'modern' views may have as much hope of *instilling hope* in their patients as they would of raising the dead, without the proper training, if there is such a thing; as some eastern religions claim as well. Voodoo followers and groups with similar beliefs currently abound in the US, and are likely to be among your patient, student, and research populations, and have yet another take on raising the dead – in the form of *zombies*. Talk about ethical conflicts in some cases.

Some religions are focused upon processes that are related to *moral, ethical or social* themes; while other are focused on *miraculous events and related saviors* and *saints*. Still others may be *light and sound* type of religions which are centered around meditation, contemplation, or even *listening for the sounds of creation* and/or supposedly being *hooked up to the sound current* by an inner teacher or one's *higher self* (51,99,100,105).

There are religious tenets that propose that spiritual salvation is based upon proponent's belief about, and accounts of, the lives of, *past spiritual leaders*; others that claim that a leader must be a *living one* and yet others that believe that a *spiritual text* can be ' *the living guru.*' (98)

There are even modern day stories of chelas (students) who claim that their teachers have 'appeared' to them after death and as solid as ever as though they had never died (116). Claims of Tibetan lamas being able to create living phantoms that appear as though they were real people, called *tulkas* (24), and are also part of your client's collective views on religion.

Oxford scholar, Evans-Wentz (29), proposes that not only are the yogic powers of the so-called 'adepts,' including teleportation and raising the body temperature, very real, but that they may be undeveloped human capabilities that are also teleological in nature; like a baby animal learning to adapt to freezing weather or the eagle soaring high in the sky in search of life sustaining food.

Some religions are based upon elaborate dress and ceremonies and some are clearly based upon *magic* in a variety of possible forms.

There are also religions that are based upon human interactions with the so-called *elemental kingdom*, including, but not limited to; elves, fairies, devas, (115) and other nature spirits including those that are claimed to be involved with the creation and operation of entire galaxies.

Still other religions are involved with interactions with common angels, archangels, and those much higher levels of angels mentioned in the spiritual scriptures throughout the world. Like it or not, still other patients and students are involved with religions that are associated with the so called 'demonic hierarchy,' and may even include animal and human sacrifice and ceremonial magic, as part of their religion. More and more of your clients may be focused upon systems based upon mystical fellowships, including the *Great White Brotherhood* (57, 58), or the Variagi Masters (105), and so forth.

I know of at least one religion that is based upon the processing of *extremely traumatic events* that are claimed to have occurred over vast periods of time in the regions of *matter, energy, space and time* and that are claimed to be recorded at both *genetic* and *spiritual* levels (47).
These traumas are said to have happened to 'us' through the evolution of a myriad of forms, including mineral, plant, animals and human kingdoms.

Serious interests in particle physics (110), astronomy, evolutionary biology and human consciousness are sure to breed many new and innovative religions that are *based more on hard scientific facts* than they are on philosophical, theological, or metaphysical constructs.

Scientists already know of at least 100 sub atomic particles that comprise the matter within 100 *billion* known star systems typical of more than 130 *billion* known galaxies (111) that make up a part of a universe which is believed to be part of a group of universes called a *multiverse* (112).

Now, lets us think of how modern views on astrophysics might be integrated with more traditional views. For example, there are many mystical texts that divide existence into three broad categories; the grouping of planes that correspond to physical existence, those that pertain to 'pure' spiritual essence and those that are a hybrid between the physical worlds and the spiritual worlds, or the spirito-material worlds (51, 99,100,105). To complicate matters further, it is commonly accepted that these more spiritual worlds are much larger and comprehensive than the billions upon billions of star filled galaxies within the physical universe. The theosophical ramifications are astronomically mind boggling.

With more than 2000 religions already officially in existence, the multi culturally savvy educator or clinician has her/his work cut out for them if they want to provide a culturally sensitive environment for their patients or those that their students may one day interact with.

A common practice in industry is to have *multicultural days* and related communications strategies. During these multicultural events, foods from different ethnic backgrounds are often provided to participants for free or at a limited cost. Innovative hospitals can help make patients happy and proud by following similar suit.

Another practice that is common in industry is the use of newsletters, online posts and posters that give a short synopsis about unique religions that employees may be a part of. With Wikipedia and other online information groups out there, the task of communicating about patient's religions is not such a daunting task these days.

Perhaps having an information 'e terminal' or written materials in interfaith chapels in healthcare settings is not such as bad idea.

When trying to understand diverse religions, it is most important to look for *core themes* that may be relevant to the *clinical population of interest*. Here are a few to think about. Please fee free to add your own themes of relevance as you become more culturally sensitive.

1) Basic tenets and history, including when the religion was started and by whom
2) Who are the major players of interest and what did they stand for, such as angels, saviors, spiritual masters, etc
3) Critical events of significance, such as healings, returning from the dead, speaking in tongues
4) *Heavens* and other *planes of existence*, including explanations in spiritual texts of diverse origin
5) Ethics, morals, and sins

6) Gender considerations regarding practitioners, interactions with other patients and family considerations
7) Food constraints, such a vegetarianism, Kosher blessings and restrictions, etc

Remember that *religious convictions* can be among the most powerful concepts known; wars have been fought over them, people have been burned to the stake because of them and buildings demolished due to disagreement about them.

I once knew a Jewish Rabbi who included a form of *energy medicine* in his spiritual practice and swore that it was a manifestation of the Holy Spirit, that it was a highly effective treatment modality and that it was harmless in the worse case.

Around the same time, I knew someone from a Christian sect who felt that forms of *energy medicine* are the work of the devil and represent evil personified. Other Christians had very positive perceptions about this very popular healing modality.

A common theme that I gathered from these and similar conversations was that there is a belief that if we are in a *state of balance* so that the holy spirit may work through us, then the person being healed is being healed by the grace of God. On the other hand, there is another common idea that if we get in the way, by *psychically* trying to direct healing energy to where we think it needs to go, then were are in essence playing with witchcraft, especially if we direct the energy without the permission of the recipient.

There are people who feel the same way about prayer and tend to pray to declare themselves to be a *vehicle for the Holy Spirit*. This is similar to saying out loud or to oneself, *may God's will be done*. While some declare that Gods will is always being done anyway, others claim that by this type of prayer, that the Holy Spirit may readily use us as to somehow facilitate healing in another.

Remember that patients want to *feel good about* what they are doing, that they can have a sense of *hope* in this lifetime, and a feeling of *confidence* and peace in an afterlife if that is in their belief system.

Since some clinicians may be more motivated by *power, achievement and self-actualization* than what is best for their patients, they may have to put their preconceived notions about what their patients are OK with aside. They may also have to ask themselves if they are planning to do what is in alignment with the patient and his/her family's *spiritual convictions* or what the clinician wants for their own benefit or for reasons related to students, residents, fellows or sales persons that may be contrary to customer requirements. Gender issues and concerns may be considerable. They may have to be reminded that 'it's not about them or their careers.'

A *customer requirements survey* can be a great way to capture things that are important to customers/patients ***before*** *they are subjected to any processes* that may be contrary to their convictions. To be effective, requirements may be broadly categorized accordingly into:

1) Critical
2) Important
3) Would like to have
4) Can live with

For example, the survey might include requirements such as:

Patient Requirements Information

Area	Requirement	Importance	Comments
Diet	Vegetarian	Critical	No eggs
Attendees	All Female	Critical	No male students, residents
Dress	Discuss	Critical	Discuss
Noise	Quite after (PM)	Important	Roomates
Outdoor	Every day	WD Like	No wheel Chair

It is important to make appropriate extended conclusions from this initial customer requirements survey.

For example, the female patient who asks for only female attendees would not want a salesman present during her colonoscopy and might want any photos taken to be restricted for modesty and kept only in area that she agrees on.

The coordinators might also include that these may also be requirements of her chosen religion and that that religion, in addition to her individual preferences, might have very strong influence over her. A *breech of religious conviction* might also put other patients under extreme stress, or put them in great danger due to possible religious retaliation, and must be taken as a potential safety issue of the highest priority. In some cases, inconsiderate treatment by the wrong person could be worse than the disease itself!

Remember, parents have gone as far as to let their children die for their religious convictions, and that many patients rather die than eat unblessed food, for example.

It is also important to keep in mind that the patient may *not be interested at all in helping you train your healthcare students, residents or fellows* and may not want them present, or to participate in procedures for many reasons, including safety concerns.

With popular press reporting a typical average mortality rate of nearly 100,000 per year, patients are taking their rights as customers very seriously these days, and may not want students or residents distracting others, let alone be performing procedures.

Of course, the importance may change with varying situations and at different times, so the questionnaire may need to be comprehensive in nature and need to be repeated often; throughout a hospital stay for instance.

Differing views on a common theme are also critically important to consider from the viewpoint of the patient, research subject or student.

For example, the Theosophical Society's take on the *Holy Eucharist* is quite elaborate and mystical in nature and is related to the planes of existence. One the other hand, while the position of the Catholic church may also be mystical in nature, the pomp and ceremony of the Catholic Mass may have lots to do with the *perceived importance* of the process on the one hand and may indeed be successful in invoking the holy spirit enter the bread of the host.

Regardless of the true efficacy of the healing oils used during the Lenten healing mass or the candles used for the *blessing of the throat*, *perceived* importance can make all the matter in the world.

So then, the perception of the client or patient regarding the *importance* of a spiritual intervention must be ascertained before the intervention is implemented.

For example, the use of *shamanic drumming* may be useful to help alleviate hypertension in the patient who not only understands the concept of *entrainment* of the human nervous system by musical rhythm; the patient must also feel good about the importance of and overtones associated with shamanism to want to participate.

What do you think the impact on the patient's blood pressure will be if they think that shamanism *is of the devil?*

So then, how the spiritual intervention is packaged is critically important for it to be successful.

Custom tailoring for individual patients may also be useful to maximize positive impact. For example, one patient may think that shamanism is cool, while another may shun the process unless the word *shamanism* or *psychic* or *energy medicine* is eliminated from the intervention package completely.

Of course, cost considerations are always an issue, and in some cases must be discussed carefully with the patient, including a recommendation to another facility that may more readily accommodate their requests.

Keep in mind that the world is getting smarter and that many patients may know more about lots of things than the clinician, researcher or educator; including the complexity of *neuroscience*.

The Neurobiology of the Soul

This chapter is designed to help the reader understand the relationships between physical world anatomical structures and what might be considered to be *higher functions*.

These ideas can be helpful for the professional who may tend to think in highly structured physical terms to think in more 'out of the box' ways.

Conversely, those who may tend to think in more 'etheric terms' – come on you know who you are!- may be prompted to think more concretely.

Ideally, the etheric and the practical sides of things will meet cognitively on common ground. The ability to switch between viewpoints is paramount to becoming more *diversity sensitive*, including multicultural and intellectual aspects of diversity.

I think that the human brain and nervous system is the epitome of all of creation in this universe. The sheer volume of cells comprising this 'engineering marvel' of nature is staggering to me, while the complexity of the system would dwarf the intelligence behind the fastest and most powerful computers on Earth. The nervous architectural schema, from the level of the ultra-minute *dendritic spine* to the most complex computational structure of peripheral and central nervous function is quite amazing indeed.

The calculus of Leibnitz and Newton, the 'seven wonders of the world,' and all fine art, music and poetry that ever was or ever could be are outputs of this most unique system. All religious ideas and every complexity of physics, chemistry, biology and medicine are among the outputs of this computational wonder programmed for survival. Each of our emotions and all of our hopes and dreams are part of this magnificent cybernetic system. Every dance danced, every play enacted and every speech ever conceived and spoken, when boiled down to its lowest common denominator, was programmed for us 'to live and evolve to our greatest potential.'

I think that the highest, the most important, and the most powerful thing that we can do as humans is to appreciate, love, honor, create, and manifest beauty. Our *sense of beauty* is our grandest perception, while its manifestation is our loftiest goal. While the perfect symmetry of a beautiful face has 'launched a thousand ships,' the *limbic systems* within our brains are striving hard to assure that our genes are carried forward by the *fittest, strongest, and most capable* of organisms.

While some may claim that the *pineal gland* is the 'seat of the soul,' and the 'eyes the windows of the soul,' the 'Godspot' within the medial *temporal lobe* may be a close contender to both. Or perhaps these two computational elements represent two poles of the same system, both focused upon different aspects of beauty, akin to the brain/mind synthesis of Plato and opposed to the body-mind dualism of Descartes and Hippocrates. *As above, so below!*

From an eastern religious perspective, humans are said to have a variety of bodies, in addition our physical bodies. Names like 'astral,' 'causal,' 'mental', and 'etheric' bodies are commonly used western terms to describe the lower ones (84), supposedly ascribed to the realms of matter, energy, space, and time. The term 'soul body' may be used by some groups (105) to describe what mystics have deemed closest to our pure essence. I think that while these concepts may be mind-boggling to the traditional western mind, the great influx of eastern docs and patients makes it important to understand their spiritual mindset. Whether modern evidenced-based medicines will ever link these higher bodies to the pineal gland is open to speculation, but fun to think about.

While we are on this line of esoteric thinking, it might also be interesting to think about the role of sleep and its relationship to the soul. Do we really travel to distant places during our sleep, as some postulate (61,105)? If so, then perhaps the production of the sleep-inducing chemical, *melatonin*, may graduate from functional neurophysiology to being an integral part of the 'seat of the soul system.' Following this line of logic, then the *reticular activating system*, (partly within the midbrain) might be considered to be part of a system that drives the soul!

While this is all speculation, and perhaps just fancy and fun, the very real human brain operates at a variety of *frequencies and wavelengths* that relate to different states of consciousness. Through modern EEG and related techniques, we now know some things that the ancients, including Kabir (20) and Rumi, did not. As we change states of consciousness, our brainwaves also change into measurable and characteristic patterns. For example, in normal waking states, we tend to have high amounts of the faster beta and some slower alpha waves dominant. As we get into sleep states and so-called higher levels of awareness, our brain wave frequencies actually get slower. These theta and delta brainwave frequencies are also characteristic of advanced meditation. Are the resonant systems within the human brain oscillating with larger cosmic vibrations? My background in electrical engineering will not allow me to discount this far-reaching possibility. There are potential pearls of wisdom everywhere and the only way that I know to shift paradigms is to really think outside of the box. It is far too easy to just move to another corner of the box!

I find it interesting that not only do long time mediators spend more time in theta and delta states, but they also have characteristically high levels of *endogenous opiods* within their brains. These elevated 'beta endorphins' are well known to be linked with a sense of wellbeing, tranquility, and a profound sense of deep relaxation.

Now back to the 'Godspot.' This very special area in the temporal lobe has been the focal point of much current research and much more speculation. There is reason to believe that when the brainwaves in this region are rapid that humans tend to feel isolated and alone. Conversely, when the God spot resonates at the slower brainwave frequencies, we tend to feel a sense of connectedness with each other and with all that is.

I think that this region of the human brain may be the *Rosetta Stone* that will open up many new vistas for the bold and adventurous neuroscientist and humanist alike. There are many questions that remain to be answered. Are there auditory pathways that are linked with the 'God spot' that make us feel a sense of spirituality when we listen to what we perceive as sacred music? What about 'sacred spaces' within the domain of human architecture or the architects of nature. Why do we feel such a sense of profound beauty in such spaces? And, why does Frankincense add to the intensity of these feelings? Are *entorhinal* and *olfactory* cortex (95) significant players in the neurobiology of spirit? Researchers involved with the use of essential scents, like lavender for relaxation, may do well by understanding the importance of the underlying cortical involvement.

I am particularly fascinated by pioneers, such as *neuropharmacologist* Candice Pert's discoveries that *neuropeptides* are present on the cells of both the brain and the immune system. She also found that there are higher levels of neuropepides in areas of the body close to those described in Hindu treatise on 'energy centers' along the spinal column (116). Current studies on the positive relationship between yoga and 'anti-stress chemicals,' like DHEA (*dehydroepiandrosterone*), have, in my opinion, expanded the concept of the 'seat of the soul' to include the whole body.

Of course, I also think that there may be some more pragmatic views to consider from within the realm of human evolution and survival. As mentioned elsewhere in this book, there is evidence to suggest that hypertensive patients may benefit from art that mimics the African Savanna or parts of the English Countryside. Characteristics of the landscape, including trees and open spaces, may be very important cues to the pursuit of food and safety and the avoidance of becoming food for some other animal also trying to survive.

I think that there is a very real possibility that a central processing center, conveniently called the 'God spot,' may respond to a variety of inputs from the senses with a universal characteristic output. The God spot's output, in the form of wellbeing, connectedness and even divine love, may very well help us to understand the sense of beauty, how beauty may be linked to survival and how the physical body and the 'soul body' may be connected! As above, so below....

Sometimes the spiritual side of patients and clinicians can get bound up in darker side of things. At these times, we may need something that can free our spirit.

Laughter, Humor, and Fun

When someone is seriously ill, laughter can indeed be the best medicine, when used appropriately, in the right way and in the proper context.

When I was in high school, a friend, also named Mike, and I, decided to skip school and hang out with another friend who had moved to another town and also decided to skip school.

The girl we had gone to visit was only 15, but still wanted Mike to let her drive his mom's car. He kinda obliged by letting her steer when he worked the gas pedal and clutch and shifted gears in the old Studebaker that was already vintage when we were teens.

He decided to scare her, so as a joke he starting applying the gas pedal to make the car drive real fast. She swiftly lost control and we all ended up hitting a stone wall head on at about 50 Mph.

The other Mike was the only one to get hurt seriously, but we all hung out in the emergency room to await his diagnosis, including broken ribs, internal bleeding and a broken nose.

While contemplating what to tell my parents, I started to hear Mike laughing from his ER cot. He was by himself, yet laughing uncontrollably. We at first thought, knowing the jokester he was, that he was laughing at our fear of telling our parents what had happened.

What was really happening was that the laughter was helping him in some *way to cope* with his injuries; his parents totaled car, and the consequences of getting caught cutting school, again.

Laughter can serve a variety of adaptive psychological functions. These functions include, but are not limited to, *stress relief* (120), panic abatement (21), and *distraction*.

In Mike's case, all three functions were at work, trying to help him deal with a tough situation. I observed a similar occurrence when he almost lost his thumb playing with fireworks.

Leiber (120) posits that, "humor can serve as a powerful mediator between stress and stress reaction, both at the psychological level and at the physical level."

The result of these psychological functions is not only adaptive from a psychological perspective; enhanced immunity, mitigation of severe pain reactions and many physical results can occur.

In one case, a famous editor, Norman Cousins, claimed that he cured himself of a very painful and often lethal connective tissue disease, *ankylosing spondylitis*, primarily by a strategic use of laughter. *

Cousins would watch amusing videos every day while in the hospital. He concluded that even ten minutes of intense laughter would allow him to sleep peacefully for several hours afterwards.

Of course, it is extremely important that the patient is:

1) OK with this type of therapy

2) Not offended by either the type and/or timing of the *laughter intervention*

3) Not in a severe crisis state when the intervention is happening

When a person has suffered a severe trauma, it is reasonable to conclude that they might not resonate with jokes, funny videos or even want to converse in any way.

* Note that he also took high doses of vitamin c, which could have worked synergistically along with the laughter therapy. Vitamin c is also used in the creation of the potentially relevant neurotransmitter, serotonin. Interestingly, vitamin c, especially when it is combines with naturally co-occurring bioflavonoids, is important for the creation and maintenance of connective tissue.

So, it may not be appropriate to commence laughter therapy until the patient is: somewhat stable, they have been assured that someone close to them is alive and safe, and that they have an inkling where they are and what has happened to them.

It is also important to consider that even if someone is unconscious, from surgery, a bad accident, or whatever, that the *amygdala* keeps recording the information said in the environment So, it is conceivable that anything said to the traumatized person may be recorded at some deep level of the nervous system (44) and that what was said may indeed be paired with the traumatic experience.

This concept is proven in the form of *flashbulb episodic memory* (92) even in much less extreme forms of trauma; such as learning about when the *twin towers* were struck on September 11, 2001 or when President Kennedy was assassinated.

Is it not conceivable that the trauma associated with a severe accident or with surgery could be even more significant for our survival; especially if the trauma was so strong as to make us unconscious?

Some believe that the laughter sometimes heard coming from someone who has just come out of anesthesia is also a stress coping mechanism of the highest order.

It is extremely important that the patient not assume that they are being laughed at.

The person who has just been electrocuted or has suffered a serious heart attack may also want assurance that laughter therapy is *not the only therapy* that they may expect.

Of course, inappropriate humor, including off color jokes, insulting, slanderous or racially oriented humor may resonate with negative emotions.

Inappropriate humor can facilitate just the opposite of Cousin's (21) suggestions that "it is useful to reach beyond laughter to all the positive emotions – hope, love, will to live, purpose and confidence …"

Laughter may also be contagious at very deep neuronal levels.

Fairy Tales and Mirror Neurons

The imagination has been proven time and time again to be a powerful healer, both directly and indirectly.

Folks have stimulated cancer controlling aspects of the immune system via a direct use of the link between higher cognitive processes and that system.

On the other hand, the imagination can provide a route of temporary escape from serious problems as we not only imaging, but at deep levels become the *confident and successful* heroes of our dreams, or movies and yes indeed *our fairy tales*.

Fairly tales, of course, have special significance in that they are or were delivered by parents in most cases. And of course, parents have learned to survive to an older age, so there are brain mechanisms built in to make us automatically want to mimic them. They in turn respond to cues, including *cuteness and beauty* (56), which make them want them to help us to survive further.

In my opinion, imagination, our built in archetypes and the teleological goal to mimic our parents may have much to do with cognitive and emotional processes related to our reactions to religions ideas. My ideas can be partially backed with evidenced based experimentation and are partly left to your imagination and creativity to ponder or experiment further.

In the 1960s book, *Psychocybernetics* (70), Maltz describes several experiments that are pivotal examples how our imaginations can help us to restructure our brains. In one experiment, three groups of participants were given the task of; physically shooting basketball hoops over a three week period, imagining shooting basketball hoops during the same time frame, or doing nothing.

At the end of the period, the groups came together to shoot hoops in a contest of sorts. Most interestingly, the group that actually shot hoops did not score better that the group that had vividly imagined making successful shots.

Imagination can be used in may powerful and interesting ways. While it is well known that creative visualization (70) has been successfully used to boost the immune system to control cancer, this powerful tool has also been used in many other practical ways.

For example, I was once a water safety instructor, with one very important goal: to teach lifeguards how to do their thing proficiently and safely. The training associated with being a trainer was no trivial task.

During a very busy time of my life, I had to get good at some very intricate maneuvers, but didn't have the time to physically practice for the grueling examination that I had to do well on to pass the training course.

As a last ditch effort, I decided to *imagine* practicing the very intricate processes in my head instead to in the pool.

To my delight, it not only worked, but my teacher had commented to me how well I did during the practical examinations.

In those days, long ago, scientists didn't know all that much about how the brain works, let alone having a deep understanding of such intricate processes as goal driven imagination. Today things are much different.

Jungian archetypes are very powerful built in exemplars which represent the ideals in human evolution and society. The perfect male, the perfect female, etc.

Not only do we consciously and unconsciously strive to personify these ideals, cues that remind us of them, and their awesome capabilities, get us to pay attention in many ways.

Whether we admit it or not, many humans live vicariously through *Spiderman*, *Superwoman*, and even *Jesus*, *Moses*, and *Muhammad*, Plato, *Hippocrates* and mother *Theresa*. They are ideal beings to many of us and at some level, knowing that they were real living beings gives us much comfort. The perception that be may *call upon them in their currently heavenly abodes* is even more comforting.

When the *ideal* beings who gave us life, and upon whom our very existence depends at the beginning of that life, it makes sense that we pay attention to what they say and do as our very survival depends upon doing just that.

Parents are very powerful drivers that shape our destiny during early *critical periods* when our very efficient brains are making connections that will influence us for the rest of our lives. Many of these neuronal connections are later pared down so that only the most important ones remain.

Researchers are starting to understand the significance of very special cells, called *mirror neurons* (56) *that* actually make us feel that we are doing what our ideals are doing!

Powerful emotions, like fear and love, on the movie or TV screen, can not only get our attention, we often feel as though we are the players, not the actors that play them.

Fairy tales not only help kids to get to sleep, no matter how outlandish they may be, there is a part of the human nervous system that *knows* that the ideal super heroes and heroines and their stories are indeed very real.

While in some of the most powerful stories, super heroes and mystical beings that are part of most every religious scripture may indeed be very real, many adults would fight to the death to support these ideas as adults even if they were meant to be myths and fables.

So the clinician, or health care facility, that may dare to go against the tenets of the patient's chosen religious system, may be perceived, consciously or unconsciously, as going against their patients very survival in their opinion.

The wrong attendee, the wrong food or intolerance towards an important religious observance or practice could indeed do much more to stress out the patient that any good that may possibly come out of a medical intervention.

It is critically important for the clinician to understand that while initial *parental imprinting* during early stages of development may have a profound influence on the patient's life, that later environmental, motivational and even physiological influences may in some cases be in conflict the earlier cybernetic program.

In these cases, *intra and perhaps inter psychic conflict* may result from opposing views.

For example, the treatment plan 'suggested' in the early life of the patient by their parents – i.e. antibiotics for the common sore throat – may very well indeed be at odds with the current values of the client, which may be perhaps take more Vitamin C along with oregano oil.

These and other conflicts between the patient's early parental imprinting and their later values are reminiscent of Freudian conflicts between the *superego*, representing parental survival strategies and those of the *id,* representing sometimes opposing views of the child or the child turned adult.

Some of these conflicts may manifest in the dreams of the patient.

Dreams and Dreaming from an Integrative Perspective

It is not uncommon for people, including patients; to have dreams about their impending illnesses or those of significant others. Dreams of death are also not uncommon and to some, surprisingly accurate. On the other hand, some dreams are symbolic in nature and many often turn out to be the opposite of what the dream is about.

For instance, I can recall several instances in which someone I know would have a series of dreams about death, just before someone they knew were to have a baby.

While many debate the validity of Jung's universal mind purview, the older I get, the more I am convinced that there is interconnectedness between living and even non living things in this universe. This connectedness is a scientific fact, not a fanciful, mystical groping for something special to be cool about.

Dreams have been of significance to priests, shaman, medicine women, healthcare people and
Scientists for as long as these 'professions' have been in existence. They can also be of extreme interest to the spiritual clinician because dreams are by their very nature multifaceted.

Modern science has evidence to support the *activation synthesis* (79, 92) *approach* to dreams. This viewpoint posits that dreams are in affect *gestalt mechanisms* that balance the effects of experiences that occur in everyday life. For example, if we were chased by a dog a couple of days ago, we may dream of experiences that include dogs, being bitten by animals, of a childhood dog that we no longer have. Many believe that activation synthesis helps in ways to balance neuronal and *psycho physiological* mechanisms that are associated with our desires and fears. Since the brain is by nature designed to be efficient, multiple parallel processes may be occurring simultaneously as a way to conserve resources.

Scientists have also determined that the brain cycles through a host of physiological states, each of which has characteristic brainwave frequencies and states of physiological arousal. [For a more thorough discussion of the psychophysiology of dreaming, the interested reader is referred to current literature on dreaming in a variety of psychology and psychophysiology texts and/or related websites.]

Since many of the brainwave frequencies and amplitudes are slow and intense, they may also be associated with increased intuition, including prophetic dreams.

While it may seem cool to associate these dream happenings with mystical experiences, and they may indeed be just that in some cases, there are several feasible scientific explanations.

For one thing, low brain wave *frequencies* with high *amplitude* are also associated with extra sensory perception and related paranormal experiences. Given that the brain is designed to be a problem solving machine, the possibility that it may obtain pertinent information via radio reception is not at all far fetched.

Given the right combination of *capacitance, inductance* and *resistance*, there are parts of the human brain that are very capable of picking up information that may be transmitted at specific frequencies from other physical systems, including other brains. At the right frequencies* an amateur radio operator may send a message clear around the world on less than one watt of energy. Nothing mystical about it and the very smart and capable engineers and scientists who figured out such things are every bit as *special* as the mystics and the physical systems can be very reliable under the right circumstances.

---

*The are a variety of ion channels in cells which may contribute to the creation of resonate circuits that are capable of picking up information from a variety of physical, biological or celestial systems.

In fact, when the *angular gyrus* of the human brain is activated, some people may feel that they have left their bodies and are viewing them as if being suspended from the ceiling.

Now, the interesting thing is that these potentially *observable* and *measurable* physiological processes do NOT in any way preclude the possibility that humans can and do leave their bodies during the dream state (61).*

The old adage 'as above, so below' may also have potential, albeit tenuous, explanations in physical science.

For example, it is quite conceivable that there are parts of the physical body that do indeed correspond with the so called *higher bodies* (105), mentioned earlier in this book; perhaps through *resonant* or *harmonic* processes.

There are also a variety of religious/mystical groups that claim wholeheartedly that there are beings whose job is to take humans out of their bodies during sleep and take them on spiritual journeys where they are taught valuable lessons (57, 58,105). Some even claim that there are schools and classes on other planes where people may learn during the dream state.

*There are some groups that also claim that humans may consciously and of their own volition leave their bodies at will (48, 105, 106)

When I finally decided to go to engineering school, I was an adult, with small kids and a responsible job. Under the circumstances, and given my poor high school math background, the prospect of doing well in the grueling math courses that are part of the electrical engineering curriculum was slim, or so I thought.

The engineering program was infinitely more difficult than any courses I have ever taken, even at the graduate level, including those in the areas of medicine, business, psychology or biology.

At first, I was quite anxious knowing that the drop out rate for even full time engineering students was typically at least 50 percent during the first year of matriculation; and primarily because of the math and math intensive courses. After getting through basic math, I had to take 6 more advanced calculus based math courses, starting with Calculus I and getting progressively more difficult.

I worked hard and did all the right things, including studying for extended periods, imagining getting As, eating super foods, exercising, meditating, doing exercises I had learned about re enhancing intuition, buying workbooks and study guides....but still I wasn't taking any chances. I would often pray before sleep that I would be taught *all there is to know* about math (and some other courses) during the sleeping hours.

Lo and behold, I was getting high 90s and 100s on a regular basis during classes and straight. As as my final course grades. Me of all people!!!

Quite a difference from my high school math grades. I almost didn't make it through basic algebra and ended up dropping high school geometry. Now I was using advanced concepts from algebra, trigonometry and analytic geometry just to be able to solve problems from much more difficult courses.

Of course there were many logical explanations, including *unconscious problems solving mechanisms* (7), for why I would wake up with answers to the most difficult problems I would try to solve, including the unassigned *advanced challenge problems* at the end of the chapters in differential equations, vector analysis, etc. My answers would often include the minutest details about how to best solve problems that might take 15 pages of equations to solve in the physical world.

During the final exam for my final undergraduate engineering math course, I found a problem with one of the questions and brought it to my teacher's attention. He promptly told me that 'I was mathematically gifted' and was wondering where I was getting my answers to the problems that were extremely difficult and that me finding his mistake was mind boggling to him. Since I had a very ill relative to deal with at the time, I was pleased at his comments but didn't realize the full ramifications of what he said until years later. I was more concerned about my dying relative.

Most importantly, math was becoming *fun*, and my successes were giving me more confidence in other courses, in which I was also getting As. I felt more capable of solving problems in other areas of my life, both consciously and during the dream state.

Besides gaining insights into human problems, I would solve all kinds of other types of problems. One time I even dreamt of a burnt component in a TV set I was trying to fix as a hobby. It turned out to be the exact component that was hidden and very difficult to find after several days of trying in the physical world. I would also dream of solutions to plumbing problems, automotive problems and you name it I would dream about, sometimes symbolically but more often I would *just know* things very clearly and very definitely. No one could BS me either. I would just know each time they might try and might just answer their lies with an 'OK.'

Much kudos to the clever researcher who has the wherewithal to either prove or disprove some of these most provocative claims and help to re categorize them from the realm or the *mystical and special* to that of *normal experience*. Fire, the wheel, the arch, radio, TV, automobiles, airplanes, and being on the moon were all once considered to be within the domain of lunatics, crackpots and yes indeed, *dreamers*.

Many patients have also been helped considerably by processes that let then have more control over their lives, including *lucid dreaming* therapies.

In some types of lucid dreaming, the patient learns to know when they are dreaming by noticing a cue in their dream. After paying attention to a cue within the dream, they may become an active participant in the dream processes, rather than being a passive observer.

The resolution of problems can be one benefit bestowed upon the proficient lucid dreamer. Other benefits may include lots of other spiritual benefits.

For instance, those who learn to *take control* successfully also learn to take *responsibility* and thereby enhance their confidence, self esteem and self efficacy.

With increased confidence, the dreamer can also unleash their creativity and have fun doing it. When all of these things are in place, the feelings of increased hope are bound to occur.

All of these benefits can raise the *emotional tone* (46) of the client and thereby help the patient to raise their physical, emotional and mental states to those which resonate with the positive and healing *spiritual states of being*.

There are also a variety of *energy fields* surrounding, interpenetrating and extending from living beings, which are considered by many to be impacted by and to impacting dream mechanisms.

Energy Medicine

The scriptures are filled with stories of healings, often times of a very dramatic nature, and sometimes under the ideal circumstances of being able to be healed at a distance.

While there can be significant controversy about whom and what is doing the healings, what is ok and what is evil, and so forth, the topic of energy medicine is a powerful one and can also be found emerging with the realm of technology.

There are also many claims about people who have healed themselves using a variety of techniques considered to be aspects of *energy medicine.*

While completing my post doctoral studies at Yale School of Medicine, I attended a conference on medical imaging at the Mayo Clinic. By coincidence, a panel of high level leaders decided to provide seminar attendees with the opportunities to ask any questions we wanted.

He decided to ask the big question. What will the medicine of the future be like? Their collaborative answer was both fascinating and surprising at the same time.

These leaders suggested that the medicine of the future would be energy based and that eventually there would be no need to see or touch patients directly. They thought that the healing system of the future would be much like that used in the TV series *'Star trek.'* Light, sound, magnetic fields, and electricity would be used to both diagnose and treat. The notion of distance healing was also reinforced by that conversation.

At the same conference, I met a researcher with Chinese roots, who conveyed another view on healing systems. During casual conversation, this gentleman spoke at length about 'chi,' the Chinese word for the innate energy present in all living beings. While his conversation included some anecdotes of an esoteric nature, inappropriate for this book, his stories were intriguing to say the least.

A good researcher will look for pearls among the dross. The search may take them to the most unexpected places to meet the most unusual people. While both social and cultural considerations will influence the practitioner, the observer will have to do her/his best to be objective, focused and open to new ideas. Above all, evidenced based research is needed. Additionally, powerful terms such as quantum mechanics need to be put into the proper perspective and context to be meaningful. The promoter of such advanced topics would need to have a real understanding of modern physics, and associated mathematics, to lend any real *credibility* to the topic.

As you may have guessed, my view on energy medicine recognizes both conventional biophysics and traditional healing systems. Since both modern technology and traditional chi are integral aspects of the 'new energy medicine,' this emerging and evolving field might be considered within the context of a *'bio/psycho/social/techno/spiritual'* model.

The broad-based model that I propose includes, but is not limited to, generic constructs related to traditional healing systems such as *Reiki*, *Therapeutic Touch* and *Mari- El* – which are for the most part non touch therapies, regardless of what the names may imply. The model also includes modalities based on conventional electrical energy, such as cranio electrotherapy stimulation and those that use light energy such as low level lasers. More conventional uses of light, such as for seasonal affective disorder can also be construed as energy medicine.

It may be surprising to many readers that Reiki is now in common practice in both hospice and hospitals throughout the US and abroad. This modality is now being used in operating suites to help alleviate pre and post operative anxiety. There is also promise that this approach may help to shorten wound healing and recovery times.

'Therapeutic touch' has also found its way into not only clinical settings, but research ones as well. For instance, there is a university based study in progress that is looking at the simultaneous impact of TT on both cancer cells and related normal tissue. This study is discussed elsewhere in this book There are indications that the 'healing energy' may be causing the cancerous tissue to die at the same time the normal tissue is being strengthened. Interestingly, the cells under study are isolated in containers.

The Mari -El system, while less well known than TT or Reiki, puts another spin on 'energy medicine.' The focus here is 'pulling out' negative experiences that are said to be lodged within the human system at a variety of levels. There is much conjecture as to how this type of healing system might actually work. At this point, it may be more useful to consider that this system does indeed work for some patients and those evidence-based researchers are hot on the trail to finding out how and why it does.

As part of my own research, and for fun and utility too, I have studied Reiki, Mari- El and Therapeutic Touch among many other healing modalities.

When I studied Mari – El I was still working in industry as an engineer, with a focus on quality assurance and reliability. Having been trained in both electrical engineering and quality science, I was well prepared to be debunk anything that I felt was bogus from any area. And believe me, try as I might, there was nothing bogus about this system that I could find. The classes were well organized, focused and informative.

My classmates included professionals from all walks of life. The course was well delivered and lots of fun. Thought you might find a couple of anecdotes of interest.

A woman in her mid twenties had indicated that she had had chronic pain in her pelvic area for as long as she could remember. After a Mari- El energy field session, she appeared to go into a deep trance. Shortly thereafter, her body started to undulate very rhythmically in sinusoidal like oscillation. She looked like a snake in motion. This lasted about twenty minutes, after which she awoke from the trance – pain free! At a refresher session six months later, she reported to the class that she remained pain free. No one touched her physically at all.

Another women complained about an ongoing shoulder pain that had lasted more than 30 years. The problem had also caused her to loose flexibility in her arm and was quite disturbing. Many years of medical and chiropractic intervention did little to help this woman. The woman also went into a trancelike state; only much deeper than the woman in the previous example.

During this session, she reported to the class that she felt as though she was in a marketplace long ago. She next reported that she felt as though she was being mugged and robbed by some thugs, who also stabbed her in the shoulder area. This experience was quite dramatic to observe, as she grimaced and acted as though she was re-experiencing real pain. Next, she was wide awake, jumped up and proceeded to rotate her arm as though had never had a problem. She remarked that she hadn't been able to do this in 30 years and that nothing she had tried had even come close to working for her.

While there is much conjecture about what was happening, that fact was that the result was swift and significant and had resulted after one short session, where she was fully clothed with very little light touch applied (as sometimes with Reiki and Therapeutic Touch). No one has to believe in past lifetimes, cellular memory or hypnotic suggestion to interpret these results.

As a former adjunct professor of human anatomy, and an instructor in psychology and neuroscience, I find nothing in my academic background that can explain these phenomena. I also have an advanced background in pathophysiology, physiology, and cell biology. Nada again.

However, I think that my background in the physical sciences, including engineering and physics, was more useful than my medical related training to understanding what was happening. Someday, elaborate mathematical models will definitively describe the interactions between the 'healing energy' fields and the human system.

Interestingly, my study of physics was not only fun and informative about how things like momentum, inertia, light, sounds and electric and magnetic fields, actually work, the implications regarding the human energy field really got my attention.

In some cases, seemingly unrelated things started to make things much clearer.

For example, I once saw a movie about how the *Tacoma Narrows Bridge,* in Washington state, was designed so poorly that is vibrated apart when the back and forth flow of the wind was at the same *resonate frequency* as the physical structure of the bridge itself.

An analogy is the tuning fork. Each fork, because of its unique shape characteristics, including length, width, materials, etc, will vibrate at very specific frequencies.

The tuning forks will send a sound wave through the air in such as way as to make the air vibrate at the same very specific frequency.

Now, similar forks that also vibrate at the same frequency may start to oscillate at the same frequency as the original fork.

In the case of the bridge, the vibrations became so intense that the bridge actually ripped apart!

Interestingly, multiples of specific frequencies may also have effected that are stronger that other frequencies.

For example, if 1000 vibrations per second (or hertz – Hz) would have a strong impact on similar physical systems, then 2000 Hz and 3000 Hz may also have a resonant effect. However, the farther we go from the original frequency, the less powerful we can expect the impact to be.

The same concept has been used in crowd control devices that may be shaped like long pipes (long pipes equate to lower frequencies) to vibrate at low frequencies that are similar to those found within the human nervous system. Based upon a similar sound canon that was invented by the French during WWII, and banned do to its cruelty, it is clear that sound can have a very powerful impact on humans.

These same principles may be found in radio and TV engineering, but in a different medium.

In the world of engineering physics and technology we may find that actual quarts crystals may be shaped in such as ways as to vibrate at very exact and repeatable frequencies to either receive of transmit radio waves over long distances.

For example, a crystal may be cut to resonate at exactly 144,567,422 Hz. Yes that is correct; the crystal is vibrating at more than 144 million vibrations every second reliably and repeatedly.

Similar technology is used to make watches, run parts of computers and are part of radar systems. Of course, technology being what it is, natural crystals have been replaced in some cases with other materials.

The implications are far reaching and deep conceptually.

For instance, *healing crystals* have been used for thousands of years in healing temples across the globe and for a variety of purposes.

Interestingly, natural pieces of quartz, amethyst, etc also have very specific and repeatable resonate frequencies. Engineers and scientists, including those from large companies have been trying for years to cut quartz at exact frequencies for very specific healing purposes.

Radionics and other specific frequency dependant healing modalities are very promising, yet in their infancy.

More esoteric aspects of physics, such as quantum mechanics, are also to be considered as aspects of *energy medicine*.

While the quantum mechanics approach has been used glibly to define these interactions, there may be more to these phenomena than particles being in two places simultaneously.

From elementary physics, we know that resonant systems, including the human body, include aspects of resistance and reactance, capacitance, and inductance. When put together into resonant circuits, human bodies can act as transmitters, receivers or both. This can be demonstrated when we come close to a TV or radio antenna. Our bodies can either strengthen or weaken the signal, thereby changing the reception.
We also know that many electromagnetic signals will diminish in relation to the square of the distance from the source. Interestingly, there is also a relationship between wavelength, frequency, signal strength and distance. Simply stated, low frequency signals may propagate over long distances with very little power consumption.

Every amateur radio operator knows that one can propagate a clear signal around the world on less than a watt of energy if the frequency is low (as in biological systems) and therefore the wavelength is long. This physical law is significant if put into perspective. The typical incandescent light bulb uses about 60 watts of energy.

So then, is there an aspect of 'distance healing' that works like a resonant radio system? While not as cool sounding as quantum mechanics, the system could also be multimodal and be inclusive of both waves and particles. The point is that it is conceivable that a transmitting human system could transmit a low frequency signal to another human clear around the world with very little energy consumption.

While there are individual differences between humans, the basic physical antenna systems of all humans are very similar. Therefore, both transmitting and receiving systems are matched resonantly in terms of natural resistance/ reactance, capacitance and inductance.

Could one human transmit a signal to all humans simultaneously? If so, then energy medicine can be placed upon a global scale that is far reaching indeed.

Some have also postulated that current radio and television systems could be used to transmit healing energy to people anywhere in the world. Again, the analog between modern technology and traditional chi is more than fanciful; it is a fact of nature and science.

Death, Dying, Bereavement and Traumatic Grief

I once had the privilege of helping to teach the lab section of a *gross human anatomy* course for a couple of semesters, in a professional school program. Interesting as that experience was, seeing all those dead bodies and body parts in various levels of dissections, on a regular basis, did indeed freak even me out at times. It was a constant reminder of the fragility of our very finite human existence, regardless of how many times we may reincarnate.

The impact on students and visitors was sometimes so extreme that they would occasionally be found passed out on the laboratory floor, would be led to vomit and would often have the leave the area after short stays; not just due to the nasty fragrances found in the lab. One might suggest that there is an *unconscious prime* (7) about being around the dead that may suggest that there is real bad danger real near.

An interesting aspect of this teleological view is that the response to the dead was notably *part dependant* in some cases, with predictable responses to certain parts; including, the face, the hands, the chest, the feet and the eyes. While the hands, feet, chest and face might have sentimental value, and removing and dissecting the human heart or making a midline dissection of the head and brain may have its moments, the reaction to removed eyeballs was the most significant response noted by me. The potential researcher might consider that at some level of the mind that if that body lost its eyes you might also be in danger of loosing yours; and without eyes, survival might be much compromised.

When I was taking my own anatomy courses, as a student, I learned an important point about what could happen when we do not understand a culture that may be important to us and may be foreign at the same time.

The first day I met my lab instructor at the lab, I didn't realize that in a Jewish facility that there must be two doors between the room containing the dead and the outside world, and that one door must be opened and closed before the other one may be. Given this clumsy arrangement, I managed to lock myself in the lab by myself for almost an hour. It was real creepy. I found myself amid lots of dead bodies, arms and lots of unimaginable stuff in all kinds of jars. Whistle I did, as though I was walking through the darkest, spookiest cemetery there is. In a way I was doing just that, or at least it felt that way.

The *feeling of being trapped* can rapidly escalate to *loosing a sense of control* and from there go from being stressed to a state of panic in the short term and forms of depression may ensue after extended periods.

As an anatomy student, I also had some experiences that 'got my attention.' On one particular occasion, the lab really made me think of the spiritual side of life.

I was often assigned to do the really tough stuff dissections, including the mid saggital section of the head, removal of the heart and this time, removal of the leg.

Creepy as it felt to take off a human leg, could you imagine what I was imagining when things started to fall of off one of the shelves at the exact moment the leg was completely severed. Things went inexplicably wrong for me and my anatomy professor that entire week. Could it be??????? Was I somehow dishonoring the dead? Who knows what his religious convictions were and of course I had wondered if he willingly or unwillingly donated his body to science or even knew what had happened to him. Anyway, lots of strange thoughts crossed my mind that week. And yes, of course I could have just been more alert to things. Perhaps?

It is also important, especially to critically ill patients, that their religious ideas and practices and those of their family, be honored and respected during their hospital stay. *They must also believe that they will be honored and respected after they are gone, or any effort to mitigate suffering may be in vane.*

Training in religious diversity is a must for anyone working with patients, including home care helpers, who have the privilege of working with the critically ill and dying. In the US alone, the sheer volume of religions may be unconceivable, while some of the practices indicative of their native cultures may seem quite foreign and even frightening to the health care provider.

Legal issues like perhaps the *death wish* of some who may want their dead bodies to be consumed by wild bird and animals, may be difficult to manage.

In some cultures, it in not uncommon to hear of a relative trying to communicate with the *soul* of the departed for several days after their death, in an effort to help them through the shock and confusion of losing ones physical body and the lifetime that they had just experienced. Many believe that their departed friends and relatives will meet a variety of beings during the transition period between lives.

The Tibetan (104) and Egyptian Books of the Dead suggest very adamantly to the reader that much of what happens to humans in the afterlife and even in future lives has much to do with what we believe will happen to us.

Some cultures believe that what happens next is a hybrid of sorts in which both the departed and a variety of possible beings, including angels, spiritual masters and even demons may be involved, along with the beliefs and efforts of the departed.

Regardless of what the dying may believe and their religious status and convictions, there are built in mechanisms that want us and our families to survive (45, 46) and even the thought of a relative dead or dying may bring on a variety of automated reactions (7).

While the importance of mourning and the acceptance of a normal bereavement period are well accepted, there are some individuals that react excessively to the death of someone close to them and for extreme periods of time in some cases.

Those suffering from *traumatic grief* (TG), may suffer from a variety of physical, emotional, and mental symptoms, long after the death of a loved one.

Innovative researchers may find the area of bereavement and TG to be particularly fruitful.

Here are some ideas that I put together awhile back that you may find potentially useful to consider spawning ideas for your research.

Note that while this section might appear to be a bit dense fore the average reader, this brief partial introduction for proposed research will give you the gist of what that research domain of spiritual medicine could be about.

I have included names along with references in this section for the reader's convenience.

The clinical and social consequences of traumatic grief are significant and diverse. Beyond the characteristic pattern of numbness, depression and recovery following normal bereavement, there are subsets of people who suffer from traumatic grief (TG) syndrome for extended periods of time; sometimes lasting for several years. During this period of TG, there is increased mortality in the bereaved due to a plethora of clinical problems including, but not limited to; cardiovascular disease, cancer, substance dependence and abuse, numbness, apathy, irritability and insomnia.

Stress hormones, including cortisol, catechlamines and histamine are particularly important factors in the etiology of psychosomatic aspects of TG. Beta-endorphin and melatonin regulation play a role in the diverse TG syndrome symptomologies and related therapies may be helpful in the regulation of these diseases. The type of pathology and severity may vary significantly among those suffering from TG syndrome, based partially on factors regarding *predisposition.*

In addition to genetic predisposition towards TG there may be significant *environmental developmental factors*, which may predispose someone to the TG syndrome later in life. Hofer (1996) has found characteristic response patterns in both human and monkey infants who have been separated from their mothers at an early age. New adaptive mechanisms are developed in response to loss of the survival benefits, which they had from their mothers. Without the food, warmth and sensory stimulation that their mothers once gave, these infants must develop novel response patterns to aid in their unassisted striving to survive. The contra-survival adaptation mechanisms gone awry are neither limited to infants or nationality.

In Japan, Furukawa et al (1998) found a significance correlation between alcohol dependence and loss of a parent, through death or separation, before the age of 16.
In a 1982 Swedish study, Mellstrom et al found significant increases in a variety of illnesses, including cancer, cardiovascular disease and cirrhosis of the liver as well as accidents and suicides.

At the other end of the cycle, there are issues regarding the loss of adaptation to excessive output of stress hormones and associated regulatory feedback mechanisms. Jacobs *et al* (1986) found a direct relationship between increased levels of catecholamine in those in bereavement or threatened loss of a spouse and increasing age. There is also evidence that cognitive patterns based on interpersonal relationships, such as unresolved marital conflicts (Blankfield 1989), may also predispose someone to TG.

It has been proposed that traumatic grief syndrome is a subset of diseases which can be classified under the umbrella of *post traumatic stress* disorder (Prigerson et al 2000). The disease also shares characteristics with *separation anxiety*, or perhaps *separation adjustment* might be an appropriate classification category. In any event, the disease has characteristics of both PTSD and separation anxiety.

It may be useful to consider biological subtypes of TG, based on occurrence and intensity of outward symptomology and individual pathology. There may be underlying biological correlates which are shared with other distinct disease entities and which are more prevalent in specific groups of TG sufferers than in others. There also appears to be distinct biological characteristics which are unique to TG. An understanding of these clusters may be crucial to focused understanding and mitigation of risk.

A proposed *'TG - obsessive type'* may have the biological tendency for *excessive rumination*, inclusive of *intrusive thoughts* of the deceased and compulsive searching behaviors. This subtype may very well share biological predisposition with the obsessive-compulsive personality type; more so than other TG sufferers.

These characteristics may include structural abnormalities with the *caudate, corpus striatum* or *cingulate regions* of the brain; or characteristic problems with *serotonergic, dopaminergic* or *histamine* regulating systems.

'TG addictive type' may share underlying biology with non-TG sufferers who also abuse, or are dependant on, addictive substances. These risk factors for this TG cluster may include, but not be limited to; abnormalities in *endogenous opiod* and *dopamine* systems and *glucose* regulation. The underlying biological predisposition may be manifested primarily as substance abuse or dependence as well as excessively long or intense numbing and associated withdrawal-type symptoms after the numbing period.

The *'TG suicidal-depressive type'* may have similar biological markers with those suffering from major depression without TG, while having features which are unique to TG. The markers for this subtype may include; characteristic problems with *melatonin regulation*, serotonin metabolism, *histaminergic* dysfunction and *cortisol* regulation and may be manifested as *apathy, antisocial behavior, insomnia* and seasonal affective symptomology. Clayton (1990) tells us that about 15% of bereaved persons experience a long-term depression. It is expected that the depressive subtype may have different DST results, which may be indicative of ineffective cortisol regulation. All of the proposed subtypes may have characteristic nutritional dependencies or deficiencies as well as *brainwave signatures* in terms of presence and intensity of alpha and beta frequencies. It is suspected that characteristic asymmetries in frontal lobe functioning in this TG subtype may be similar to those suffering major depression and different than other TG sufferers. The answer to this question, through functional imaging or EEG studies, may eventually lead to understanding the differences in brain function between major depressive types and the TG subset of PTSD.

An evolving *assessment strategy* is proposed to better understand the biological etiology and morphology of traumatic grief. The initial assessments will be directed at understanding biological manifestations of the most significant factors in the mortality of the TG sufferer; including cardiovascular disease and immuno-suppression associated with cancer. A comparison with other related diseases syndromes, including major depression without TG, PTSD, and OCD is recommended either initially or for consideration for future studies. Of course, assessment without intervention doesn't directly alleviate suffering associated with the TG syndrome.

Intervention proposals are grouped into two broad categories; basic bio-behavioral and future innovations. The first group is focused on exercise and relaxation therapies and the second group consists of a broad array of possible innovations in the field. These considerations for the future include, but are not limited to; *cognitive therapies*, *resolution of traumatic memories*, *imaging*, *electrophysiological* innovations and specific *nutritional* considerations. They are included here since there are relationships with the initial assessments and interventions. Due consideration needs to be given to the allocation of resources associating their viability and feasibility. It is recommended that these activities be done in concert with the implementation of other potential initial assessments and interventions.

The initial interventions could be directed towards *exercise* and *structured relaxation techniques*. Physical exercise is known to induce *beta-endorphin* release, which may be associated with decrease in alcoholism, enhanced feeling of well being and weight regulation. These expected outcomes have both psychological and physiological benefits, such as; improvements in cardiovascular health as well enhanced self-esteem and self-efficacy. Social interactions will be encouraged.

The second aspect of the initial intervention strategy is focused on structured relaxation techniques targeted at the reduction of *catechlamines* and *glucocorticoids* and the morphology and symptomology associated with their excess.

Additional future interventions may include those targeted on *cognitive restructuring*, the *resolution of traumatic memories* and additional specific *nutritional* intervention plans. While current and future drug therapies may be indicated or may evolve out of these studies, it is important to recognize that among the hallmarks of the TG syndrome are the tendencies *for social withdrawal and substance abuse*. While drug intervention may be indicated in some cases of TG, all proposed drug therapeutic plans must take these idiosyncrasies quite seriously to avoid the potential for **causing serious additional harm** *to the TG syndrome sufferer and their families*.

The incidence of cardiovascular problems is greater in those who meet the proposed criteria for TG. For example, Prigerson (2001) has reported a 10.4 times greater risk of high blood pressure for bereaved meeting criteria for TG. Such high risk imposes a potentially huge socio-economic burden and must therefore take a high priority in a study of the biological aspects of traumatic grief. The link between the prolonged stress of TG and associated cardiovascular breakdown has both direct and indirect connections.

It is well known that the incidence of cancer and other indicators of reduced immune function are prevalent in those experiencing traumatic grief. Nineteenth-century physicians working with cancer patients have commonly reported cases of severe loss and grief prior to the manifestation of the neoplasm (Biondi etal 1996). There is evidence that these and other indications of immunosuppression are mediated by stress hormones; especially cortisol. This interaction is supported by investigations in molecular biology, which have discovered numerous *receptor sites* for stress hormones directly on the surface of a variety of immune system cell types. The normal physiological function of cortisol on the immune system is suppression to avoid destruction of normal tissue by prolonged immunoreactions. Over production of cortisol, and extended release periods, can have profound immunologic implications through suppression of *prostaglandins*, *thrompoxanes* and *leukotreines*.

Cortisol also inhibits the recruitment of circulating leukocytes by interfering with the vascular mechanisms associated with their attraction. Phagocytic and bactericidal mechanisms are inhibited by the suppression of neutrophil effectiveness and leukotriene stimulated respiratory bursts associated with enhancement of these immune processes. Associated inhibition of fibroblasts dampens chronic inflammatory responses to tissue injury, while thymus-derived lymphocytes, such as T-cells including helper T4 cells are also inhibited. Interleukin 1 and 2 as well as *interferons* are also suppressed by cortisol.

The mechanism of suppression is through cortisol induced *lipocortin*, a *phospohprotein* that inhibits the activity of the enzyme *phospholipase A2*. Phospholipase A2 in turn inhibits *arachidonic acid* binding, which is a precursor to *prostaglandins*, *thrompoxanes* and *leukotreines* and therefore reduces their synthesis, as a rate limiter.[*]

The astute clinician or researcher best keep in mind that those suffering from traumatic grief may simultaneously be suffering from other forms or trauma in addition to perhaps other sources of maladaptive stress; the cause of more than 90 percent of ALL illnesses.

---

[*] See Prigerson and Jacobs (2001), "Perspectives and Care at the Close of Life: All the Doctors Just Suddenly Go," for extensive overview of traumatic grief and epidemiological details

Anxiety and Depression

Anxiety and depression can become so debilitating to some people that I like to consider them to be among the *spiritual diseases*, because they can take over a person's perceptions, their personality and their social interactions. In some cases, patients become so *reactive*, versus proactive, that they become obsessed with the objects of their problems.

It is very difficult to consider spiritual issues when a client is depressed or anxious. Conversely, spiritual issues can be a primary source of these negative moods. These mood issues may also be co morbid with other problems, including, but not limited to: substance abuse, borderline personality and schizophrenia.

There has been a great deal written about anxiety and depression in the professional and popular literature, so I recommend that you brush up on the basics from a good text on abnormal psychology; preferable one that is based upon a bio.psycho.social.techno.spiritual model, with due consideration for individual differences, age, gender, culture and most of all, environmental stressors. The DMS will also give you the basics in a standardized and popular format.

In brief summary, some of the causes of these states include physiological, teleological and psychological factors interacting as parts of the human system; the patient as a composite human being.

In this abbreviated section, the focus will be upon some more advanced ideas that may point you in a more comprehensive direction, now or in the near future.

For the researcher, the potential factors and confounds associated with the states of anxiety or depression are significant. The clinician or educator must consider many factors pertaining to the etiology or morphology of these disease states; perhaps they are not diseases at all, but warning signs that real or imagined danger is near?

Many modern researchers believe that anxiety and depression are *goal directed* vestiges from earlier times in mammalian evolutionary history.

In one popular view, some forms of depression are considered to be programmed by nature to make grazing animals slow down after long period of grazing; to conserve resources by forcing resting when the likelihood of successful foraging is less at the end of the day and to get the grazing animal to be quiet and still to avoid being a target for predators. It is also conceivable that depression that is triggered by periods of darkness may also be nature's way to get animals and humans to slow down.

The conservation of resources idea can also spawn other views about why nutritional deficiency and dependency can so rapidly lead to depression or anxiety. Is it possible that when important nutrients are becoming scarce that nature, sensing disaster, may at times try to get us to slow down *to conserve resources*? On the other hand, could some of our anxiety be causing us to pay attention or be more *vigilant* about the pending nutritional disaster? Yes!

Anyway, when we initially feel trapped, for example having a roommate that doesn't pay their share of things, our initial response is to feel anxious, stressed and perhaps to have enough energy to *fight back*. The associated *anger* can also be natures of giving us enough energy change out destiny.

However, after an extended period of the roommate working on again and off again, getting fired, blaming the boss for his incompetence, making up nonsense, we may feel that we are indeed trapped.

After a prolonged period of feeling that we are trapped, the stress may become escalated to depression as a survival mechanism from our distant past.

Ever hear of a trapped rabbit succumbing after they feel that they have no chance of living. Well, humans do the same thing.

When they feel that the situation is *hopeless*, at some level of their being, they may feel that they are indeed better off dead than fighting a losing battle.

At that point, even the best meditation programs, *cognitive therapy* programs, light therapy, fitness programs, b-vitamins, vitamin c, magnesium, zinc and protein and carbohydrate of tryptophan induced serotonin production may not do the trick.

Those who prescribe antidepressants must also seriously consider that some medications may actually speed up the dying process, through side affects related to the accumulation of nor epinephrine in the synaptic cleft.

While they once just thought about suicide, the once depressed person may now have the energy to finish the trip to 'heaven.' Or perhaps the prospect of going to hell is stopping them from killing themselves.

I once had a relative who contracted a rare heart problem after getting a rare infection in a foreign island. To his shock, his heart was destroyed and he was in need of a transplant at a relatively young age.

He become so depressed that someone decided that he should have a popular antidepressant drug. Within weeks he jumped in front of a train.

At the funeral I was told that his real body was in four pieces and that he *looked so good* because he was pieced together with cardboard!

When I mentioned the story in one of my psychology classes, a young lady in the first row almost burst in tears.

She said that her brother had hung himself after taking the same drug not too long ago. He was only 24 years old.

I got the impression that there were family/social issues that needed to be worked out, and that *behaviors* associated with nutrition, fitness and perhaps cognitive approaches may have saved this young man's life.

At some level his depression went away, but at another level his sense of hopelessness was perhaps stronger than ever.

Modern technological innovations, including *biofeedback* and home *electrotherapy stimulation, music* and *brainwave entrainment* devices have in some cases been extremely helpful in balancing brain mechanisms, including *serotonergic* mechanisms.

Some fitness regimes have been found to be at least as effective, and in cases much more effective than, any antidepressant medications.

However, keep in mind that the mom who has had her child taken away or girlfriend who stays under the control of her anti social boyfriend is unlikely to be helped by *ANY* physiological treatment until these issues are resolved once and for all; often by disconnecting completely from the perpetrator.

In those cases, the patient may miraculously be healed from *spiritual suppression* and related diseases as she gets to once again live with her long lost daughter or she finally gets the nerve to throw her controlling psychopathic boyfriend out.

Those who are in any ways performing illegal activities or are in any way involved with them may be anxious for some very good teleological reasons.

The fear of being arrested, going to jail, or being killed as part of a drug transaction or a police action, is a very real and very rational reason for being anxious.

When she has felt that she has lost control over important situations like the ones described, no amount of Prozac, exercise, nutrition, or electrotherapy, or psychotherapy, is going to fix the depression.

Ask about these social possibilities first and nothing else at all may be needed, except perhaps a new place to live, a new job or schooling.

Conversely, treating the depression without losing the psychopath in her life might only speed up her death in some cases, while doing nothing but moving the locus of control further away from the person and thereby exacerbating and prolonging a hopeless situation.

Hope, Despair & Learned Helplessness

The crux of spiritual medicine in clinical practice is to remove a sense of *despair* and impending doom - better yet to create a *safe space* and a sense of *confidence* where the patient may, realign the *lower bodies* and to remove the negative emotions themselves - and replace those emotions with a sense of *hope*. Sometimes a perceived connection with a *higher power* will make the patient have more *confidence* that: the outcomes in this world will be positive and/or that the perceived outcomes in the afterlife will also be favorable.

In order to instill this sense of confidence in a higher power, many people will align themselves with the tenets and activities associated with a religion. Some patients will take things that they resonate with from several religions and/or mystical organizations and/or follow their own views as well.

Pricilla Presley, wife of the late and great king of rock and roll, once disclosed to the public that Elvis had a very deep spiritual side that went beyond his wonderful *gospel music*.

She went on to tell of an anecdote about when someone asked him why he was wearing a Native American jacket top, a crucifix, and a Star of David all at the same time. His answer was that he "wasn't taking any chances!!!" As I recall, Elvis also studied a variety of metaphysical systems, including *Theosophy* and *Self-Realization Fellowship*.

I think that the astute clinician, educator and researcher must consider that the person may be taking the same position as they *seek for hope in* an attempt to *mitigate despair*.

Bandura (6) has proven time and again, that activities that promote *increased confidence* in patients are critically important to their wellness and successes at all levels.

These confidence building activities can in turn spawn feelings of *self-efficacy (*the perception of being capable and productive*)*, which will in crease *self - esteem*.

Confidence in oneself as well as confidence in a possibly chosen care provider are the building blocks towards turning the patient away from *despair* and towards *hope*.

In cases where the patient has an addictive personality, such as in substance abusers, great caution must be used to avoid facilitating unnecessary and counter productive dependence on the practitioner. Gender considerations must also be seriously considered even in cases of talk therapy.

Many rehab centers have taken the position that in cases where therapy is useful that group therapy is commonly the therapy of choice over individual therapies, in part to avoid *dependence* issues.

Glasser's views are in alignment with those of Bandura. The primary postulate associated with his *reality therapy* (36) is that "patients are not irresponsible because they are sick, they are sick because they are irresponsible."

The combined views of Bandura and Glasser can be instrumental in the development of the most successful rehab centers.

A focus on career development has proven to be a most successful form of 'non-therapy' for many with addictive personalities. The most productive centers that I know of are concentrated on the creation of productive small businesses that are run by former addicts.

In some cases, like in the *Delancy Street foundation* in San Francisco, career development strategies include partnerships with a variety of vocational schools, colleges, graduate programs and professional schools.

A similar scenario exists in cases of chronic illness and its treatment.

Unfortunately, the patient who has failed in life many times may be suffering from one of the most difficult issues of all to deal with, *learned helplessness*. These folks may feel that they have lost a sense of control over:

1) Their illness
2) Their finances
3) Their children

These can also be the folks that are bent on making themselves fail, no matter how much someone tries to help them.

The:
1) The mother who purposefully drives without car insurance
2) The former narcotics addict who chooses to hang around others who are sure to be arrested
3) The woman who stays with the boyfriend who continuously rips off her child

have learned at some level of the brain to fail; and fail they will, regardless of what may be done for them.

Another classic example of bringing on their own self destruction is the person who will spend excessively, regardless of how much they may earn. These people will be found wasting money on needless articles that they often neither want or need. They will hold on to them, only to donate them at a later time; and then complain that they have no money; a *self imposed state* of despair and hopelessness.

They may be suffering from the *depressive* symptoms of low motivation, passivity and indecisiveness (79) on the one and can't get out of a rut. But they really can.

They may also be exhibiting the self destructive/risky symptoms of *borderline personality* (92) on the other hand

Odd at it may seem to some readers, many of you modern day US patients really believe that their troubles are caused by the *dark forces*.

The Dark Force

In a variety of cultures, there is a prevalent theme in which illness, especially those with emotional and/or mental aspects are caused or influenced by voodoo, the evil eye, poltergeists and other nefarious beings.

Many patients in US health care systems have similar viewpoints, which regardless of the clinicians' views, or any other contrived logic, are nonetheless very real to them.

Is the dark force real? You bet it is if you believe that it is; and even if you don't believe in the dark force, there is startling evidence to suggest that it may be much more than in the imagination of gullible people and lunatics. Can you really prove otherwise, beyond a shadow of a doubt?

When I was in high school, a friend and I decided to walk home after a dance. When we got near our school, we both sensed something but both of us kept real quiet. We both saw the same thing which we later confirmed. First one ghostly figure walked slowly across a playing field, and then another joined it and then two more. As we watched in amazement, the 'family of ghosts' or whatever they were that we both saw, did their thing for about ten minutes and then disappeared quietly into a wooded area nearby.

In the same area, another friend, who lived in an old house built in the 1600s reported things flying off shelves, and even that a house fire was somehow caused by mischievous ghosts.

Many folks report that chairs rock, that they see strange bright beings during the night and so forth.

Well, for one thing, energy cannot be created or destroyed under normal circumstances in this world, so it would not be too shocking to discover that dead folks may be hanging around for some reasons.

Whether they are real or not, they are sometimes things that may play heavily on the minds of some patients, and can be a source of fear and concern beyond the normal experience of most people in modern, industrialized countries.

I know a very educated and articulate nun who witnessed an exorcism in Rome. Her explanation of the details was a very convincing example of the possibilities.

The Roman Ritual, the official test of exorcism of the Catholic Church, has been around for hundreds or years and is still taken very seriously today.

Of course, demonic obsession and possession do indeed mimic psychiatric illness, which is often ruled out by psychiatric evaluation prior to the consideration for exorcism.

In this most interesting section, I would like to include more anecdotes that may be of interest to some of you. I will leave it to the reader's discretion, intuition and common sense to interpret these vignettes in their own way. I'll start with something that happened to me long ago as a teenager.

I once knew some folks who were affiliated with a *humanistic psychology* club who decided to study some occult activity in the area.

One night one of my roommates decided to host an event at our place for the fun of it, and I decided to attend. To my amazement, an English professor in attendance was a trance medium, who was accompanied by a real honest to something warlock. As a teen, I thought that this 'fortunate' event was real cool and I, being the curious young man that I was, egged them on that night, including asking for a séance.

Right before the séance, however, we had dinner and set aside some time for some social interaction. That night, I heard one of the most incredible stories and decided to call the warlock on a claim that I thought was total BS. He claimed that he had a way to get energy out of electricity. Between the laughter that I tried hard to hold back, I told this mysterious gentleman that I would be right back.

In the meantime, I went to my room to get a cord from my lamp. I carefully cut the wire, stripped insulation off the ends, plugged it in and tapped the two ends of bare wire together to make a spark, proving that the current was passing through the wire. Lo and behold, this mysterious gentleman proceeded to hold the bare wires in his hand - for real!!! - and for more than a minute. He then *got my attention*. I then asked the couple if we could have the séance in my bedroom around the *spool table* in my bedroom.

Shortly after the medium/professor started the séance, she appeared to go into a trance and began to talk about some events that had occurred long ago on the property where the present house stood.

While talk about a supposed murder that had occurred long ago, and a trapped spirit were kinda interesting, they weren't quite cool enough for a wild kid in the room – me! So, I foolishly asked if we could somehow spice it up a bit, and the warlock asked me if I was sure that that was what I *really* wanted. "Yup," was my reply.

The warlock next proceeded to recite some very strange words and within literally seconds, the temperature felt like it had dropped 20 degrees and the room started to feel real creepy.

For a minute, I felt like the cowardly lion in the *Wizard of Oz,* when he told us how much 'he did believe in spooks.' I did too that night.

I was sacred like never before, and started to pray to myself to Jesus and Mary ... like I never prayed before!!!! Then shortly, the room returned to a normal temperature and we were all back to a normal state of mind.

We were then asked, by the warlock, what we experienced, in true academic fashion.

Another attendee also felt the extreme chill in the room and proceeded to tell us that he had seen a green thing around each of us and then sensed a feeling of *extreme peace* as what he described as a miniature version of the *Virgin Mary* appearing in the center of the table.

When it was my turn, I told of how I had prayed and of how scared I was.

The Warlock proceeded to tell me how 'I shouldn't do that as it would surely ruin it.'

Ruin what??

Well, he said that high vibration beings, like Mary, would NOT allow the spirits of the dead ... to enter the room.

For weeks he tried in vane to get me to join his 'group.'

~

Shortly thereafter, a group of college girls tried to get me to join their *coven*, but something warned me not to for several reasons, which in part I was to find out real soon.

The witches told me that their *next assignment* was to collectively put a *death spell* on one of the girls parents because they had imposed a curfew on the teenage and she thought she should be able to stay out later! Yikes!

~

Many years later, I had heard a story from a Catholic priest that also 'got my attention.' This interesting gentleman told of how he was assigned to a certain part of Connecticut to help out with some serious spiritual trouble in the area, including satanic witchcraft.

Some of the groups in the area threatened to kill him for interfering with their religious activity.

~

Shortly thereafter, I heard a story about how a young woman, who had numerous problems, had stumbled upon a medal on a hiking trail. She was utterly shocked when she had realized that it was a medal of *Satan*, and swiftly threw it to the ground. Then she was even more shocked to see a very sinister man, dressed completely in black, pick up the icon and dash away through the woods.

Years later, she was guided to live in the same general area, as though it was pre planned somehow. Once, when walking her dog, she saw a man dressed completely in black rapidly approaching. In a flash he just disappeared, like in the movies, but in real life.

Another gentleman claimed that a whole black car with a very sinister looking driver, that looked somewhat like a skeleton, had the same 'vanishing fate' in the same general vicinity.

The women mentioned earlier had also mentioned seeing pentagrams and devil faces written on walls in the area, just as she might arrive for an appointment somewhere.

~

Around the same time period, I was teaching a class in psychology and asked students to share real Halloween stories if they had any.

A young man disclosed a story to the class that was so gruesome that I decided to verify what he was to tell me, and did so.

A young woman, part of a satanic group, had a baby in a local motel and then proceeded to help sacrifice the young baby in a wooded area in the vicinity.

To my utter disgust, the group apparently roasted the baby, ate its flesh and drank its blood.

I was to find out that a similar event had occurred about 10 yrs previous in a town about 20 miles away.

~

Recent to the publishing of this book, a local drug bust was the scene of a satanic ritual which had occurred in SW Connecticut. When the cops arrived on the scene of the marijuana bust, they were to find satanic writings on the walls, written in blood. They also found a human skull that was apparently used in the satanic rituals.

~

A couple of weeks later, two more human skulls were found in a nearby cemetery. This time the names of several people were found within the skulls and written in bloody cloths.

~

Shortly thereafter, the body of a dead two year old was found in a river in New Jersey. The body which was traced to a grave in Connecticut was allegedly to be used in a satanic ritual, when the attempt was foiled.

Interestingly, the newspapers had disclosed that the grave had been completely sealed, and only by a serious of coincidences was the exhumed body found, two states away. When the grave was opened, sure enough it was empty to the shear shock of the parents.

~

Switching gears and now wearing my psychology hat, I am reminded of a doctoral course I had taken in *multiple personality disorder* (MPD) and disassociative states.

Interestingly, *satanic ritual abuse* is among the most frequent causes of multiple personality disorder.

It is suggested that the severe trauma in some of these cases, often made worse by the drugs used in the rituals, can make such an impact that each personality is somehow isolated from the other personalities.

This phenomenon is akin to how the physical body may encyst infectious materials in an attempt to keep the diseases from spreading.

The astute clinician, researcher and educator may very well be aware of the etiology of MPD, including genetic predisposition, however multicultural considerations may be significant.

The spiritual healer must also consider the disease from a *multicultural* perspective.

In some cultures, for example, the practice of these rituals may not only be tolerated, they may actually be 'the thing to do.'

The thoughtful researcher must take these social factors into careful consideration to avoid potentially significant confounds. The educator may consider the broad bio.psycho.social views regarding MPD as only complete when these social factors are integrated within the curriculum.

The fact that the abusers themselves may be family members or close friends may confound the case further. Due consideration must also be given to the fact that abusers are often those in positions of considerable power, including physicians, police and government officials, etc, The implied breech of trust must also be considered both practically and academically.

The belief system of the patient may also be such that they have strong beliefs in a systematic and extensive *demonic hierarchy*. This hierarchy, often alluded to in religious scriptures, may include many levels and can be considered to be the 'anti' version of the angelic hierarchy, with its *Powers, Principalities, Archangels*, and so forth.

~

Soon after the death of a relative, I was in her 18th century house with some relatives. While we all felt that for some reason we were not alone, one of my relatives felt particularly uneasy.

Since she was also the family photographer for this outing, she took a few interesting pictures within this uniquely beautiful antique home.

Lo and behold, the picture in the room where we all felt 'something,' was full of orbs, little globes of light, sometimes considered to represent ghosts.

While there were many other possibilities, like link or dust on the lens, moisture…the really odd thing was that she took and retook several pictures through the house and only in that most interesting room did the orbs appear.

About four years later, I had the opportunity to talk with a very unique and in tune real estate lady. This very devout Christian woman had picked up on the very same things that I and my family members picked up on in the past; but this time not only in the main offending area as before, but also included other areas of the house.

When she was given permission to pray in the *name of Jesus*, one could actually feel a lightness and happy feeling about the house

While one might argue that *suggestion* was in place and there was no real healing - it just seemed that way-, or that Moses or Krishna had similar capabilities or that the whole things was a bunch of crap, the nice feeling remained and the gloomy feel of the old house was gone as far as I was concerned.

In some Native American cultures, the use of burning herbs, including Sage, have been used traditionally for millennia to clear places of evil influences.

In other traditions, the use of quartz or amethyst crystals and/or the aroma of lavender have been used for similar clearing rituals.

The use of lavender essence has been applied to warm computer monitors in more modern healing traditions - in the workplace.

So then, dear readers, is it reasonable to conclude that even dealing with the so called *dark force*, can be a multi dimensional processes with the potential of being applied as a bio/psycho/social/techno/spiritual healing system?

You bet it is; and you can also bet that the researchers out there can, and will in the near future, apply *multi factorial* experimental designs to legitimate studies of the dark force.

If you care not to respect the patient's spiritual philosophy, even if it is way out there in your opinion, or even evil from your viewpoint, remember it's *not about you,* or how smart you may think you are.

Use great caution if you are <u>really</u> smart!

A spiritual advisor must be religion savvy too.

Stress and Chronic Disease

Excessive and non-productive stress is one of the most important public health issues on our planet, costing more than 200 billion dollars annually (41) in the US alone. More than 50 percent of all medical visits (19), about 80 percent of all workplace accidents (91), and millions of lost workdays have been attributed to excessive stress. Nearly 100 million people in the US take medication for stress and the lost opportunities attributed to excessive stress are socially and ethically relevant to the highest degree.

In this abbreviated chapter, I plan to share some of my views on the neuro-pathophysiology of maladaptive stress and some related social ramifications. Excessive stress can be caused by social factors, while it may also lead to social problems. I think that the healthcare provider of the present, as well as future providers can find no area of study to be more important to her/his practice than 'stress leadership.' Of course, a leader is someone that people are voluntarily willing to follow, is focused upon prevention, and is often perceived as a teacher.

The 'stress leader'/physician of the future will be adept at not only preventing stress-related illnesses, but will have a keen grasp on both its etiology and morphology. I think that this humanitarian of the highest degree will, if trained properly, follow a bio/psycho/social/techno/spiritual model and her/his patients will benefit greatly from this approach.

The 'human side of healthcare quality' will be a broad-based approach where psychological and social factors will be duly considered along with the biological ones. Intelligent uses of science and technology can be important aspects of multi-factorial stress leadership designs. However, inclusion of spiritual considerations will provide well-rounded approaches towards stress related disease processes and the human beings impacted.

I believe that human based practices can be the only effective ones, and that a deep understanding of underlying human pathophysiology is an important part of the equation. A *multi-dimensional system can be the only true holistic one and would include factors with are both genetic and environmental in nature.*

The humanitarian/stress leader will need to know how and why initial sympathetic excitation can readily escalate to pituitary-mediated release of adrenal stress hormones in an attempt to 'prepare for battle' or take flight. I think that a clear understanding of the biochemistry, physiology, and pathology of chronic disease associated with prolonged stress is well worth the effort.

From the psychobiological perspective, the curiosity of a healer-scientist cannot be better exercised than by understanding stress-related pathophysiology. Some may be intrigued by the intricate connections between sensory inputs and both cortical and sub-cortical structures within the 'stress cascade.'

I am certain that a deep understanding of hippocampal and amygdala based memory systems could shed light on many new and important steps in our understanding of stress related trauma and how to deal with its effects. The importance of memory formation occurring during severe trauma, including the 'surgical memory,' can shed insights of considerable social relevance.

The successful physician of the future will also understand stress-related relationships between the immune system and the nervous system. I suspect that the important field of psychoneuroimmunology (86) has yet to reach its full potential in our understanding of neoplastic (cancer) and infectious disease processes and their progression. What greater understanding can those with this mindset have than to truly understand the reciprocal relationships between the neuron and the cells of the immune system?

For example, it is now known that both neurons and immune cells have receptor sites for neuropeptides and neurotransmitters. A pragmatic understanding of how and why excessive stress hormones may weaken immune function is of considerable social relevance. Conversely, secretions from immune system leukocytes have influenced the growth of neuronal structures and may even play a role on how we 'remember' our illnesses at very deep levels.

The biological and psychological aspects broached are only part of the 'human stress-strain system.' Thwarted intrinsic motivation, coupled with a variety of social complications, may be the missing link to a considerable amount of baffling and chronic disease processes, including some gastrointestinal (31) and endocrine ones. The stresses produced by these often-overlooked factors can produce life-threatening strain within the human organism. Meditation, fitness, and exercise are rapidly becoming the treatments of choice, among even the most conventional of practitioners. But these wonderful approaches are not enough!

Maslow's *hierarchy of needs* (92), while being simplistic in nature, illustrates another piece of the broad-based stress-strain system that *all* responsible practitioners would surely be interested in. We all have needs, beginning with the most basic such as for food, shelter, and security. Once these basic motivators are fulfilled, our social needs become paramount, followed by those associated with self-esteem. Finally, at the top of the hierarchy, is our need for self-realization.

When any of these needs are thwarted along the way, there is a dissonance between what we perceive that we 'need' and the fulfillment of those needs. This stress scenario can become much more complicated when our expectations are not realized. In my opinion, these unfulfilled needs can cause *severe* and even life threatening stress when we perceive that we are being treated inequitably. Even the most powerful drugs, or the most well meaning 'pseudo-holistic' stress management regimes, may not be enough. This is part of what cardiovascular disease and cancer live on, while ironically being the least understood aspects of the stress-strain system! In the worst case scenario, the complications of unresolved extrinsic conflict can potentially bring the patient over the edge.

Diet, exercise, and relaxation processes can do wonders when intrinsic and extrinsic conflict is managed simultaneously. Either approach by itself is only a partial solution, considerably less effective than the sum of both approaches working in harmony.

I think that any doctor, nurse, or allied health care professional can benefit tremendously by understanding the social dynamics of the human stress-strain system.

From a broad based 'technical' perspective, the human stress-strain system can only be managed in ways that are suitable for the unique patient, including practitioner/patients. For example, those who need to be cooped up inside may benefit greatly from important contributions within the living environment itself. Full-spectrum lighting (119) and natural light transmitting windows and skylights can do wonders during the winter months. Innovative uses of art, color and music can be among the most important considerations in minimizing environmental aspects of stress. For some folks, the creation of art itself may do much to relieve tension. In fact, I think that pursuing these activities may even help to strengthen our immune systems in ways yet to be discovered!

Proper air ionization (the electrical charge present in the air itself) can also do wonders for overworked patients (9). The abundance of negatively charged air is one of the reasons we feel so great in pine forests (negative charges are emitted through sharp points like those found in pine needles), on mountaintops, and at the seashore. Negative ion generators, indoor water falls, and even properly placed plants can change the electrical characteristics of the air itself towards harmonious human existence.

I think that the stress-strain system, including its underlying neural structures and biochemical cascades, can only be understood completely by understanding multicultural diversity and spiritual aspects of the overall human system. For example, the well meaning and innovative clinician can even cause significant stress by prescribing diets that are not in alignment with the individual's cultural and religious background. Even the choice of the practitioner her/himself may contribute in a variety of ways to stress of the patient if social and cultural aspects are not carefully considered (68).

From another angle, hope, trust, and a sense of being in alignment with something of spiritual significance can do much to prevent or alleviate stress. At a deeper level, all of the stress and strain management considerations discussed may have focal points of interest within the human system itself. For example, I think that the little understood 'God spot' within the medial temporal lobe of the brain (80) may have much to do with how we process many stress-relieving approaches discussed. This includes art, music, meditation, biofeedback, and prayer. Our perception of cozy and inspiring architecture may help us to feel 'de-stressed' when this spot vibrates at lower brainwave frequencies.

I believe that even the choice of literature and poetry, including that with spiritual significance, can have significant and even perhaps measurable impact regarding its impact on the human stress-strain system. There is a vast area of untapped potential between the areas of neuroscience and the arts and humanities that can do much to alleviate stress related disease.

I strongly believe that 'stress-strain' related mechanisms are behind a great many chronic diseases. Broad-based considerations for intrinsic and extrinsic conflict are major factor in much of this disease.

Ethical and valid use of the sciences, technology, and spirituality will provide great benefits if framed within the context of multicultural diversity and human value systems. Innovative uses of the arts and the humanities are sure to play significant roles as our understanding of human stress and strain continues to evolve.

Without due consideration for nutrition, even the best stress leadership approaches are doomed to failure.

~ Clinician do no harm. Note that your very presence, in some cases, may do more harm than good. It's not about you! ~

Nutrition, Fitness and Spiritual Wellbeing

In this Earth world, for most people spiritual medicine is focused upon creating a *healthy vehicle for spirit to manifest through*; albeit there are those extraordinary folks who claim to be able fix physical things from a higher mental/spiritual level and some who even claim to be able to operate their physical bodies while existing as spiritual beings outside of the body for the most part (48,105). Even these *strange propositions* are all things that the spiritual medicine enthusiast is best to know about if they want to really understand the complexities of modern cultural diversity. Most of all, these ideas are what some of your patients, students and research subjects believe in.

Proper nutrition is first and foremost and proper nutrition means many things to those whom you may be working with or trying to better understands. Some groups are dead fast against the eating of ANY *animal products*, while some will only eat foods that are *blessed* by a spiritual representative from their religious clergy. *Gluttony* is considered to be a sin in many faiths and ritual *fasting* is considered mandatory in many groups.

There are generic aspects of human nutrition that are germane to spiritual manifestation in the mundane world regardless of one's faith.

Most people need a *balanced diet* to maintain a healthy and appropriate vehicle for spirit. The proper amounts of protein, carbohydrate, fatty acids, vitamins and minerals, and water, *regardless of the forms they come in*, are necessary to development and maintain a healthy and functioning nervous system (83) - through which their higher cognitive and spiritual aspects may manifest through.

It is also important to understand that many unhealthy habits, including drinking excessive alcohol, can create *deficiencies*, especially in those with genetic *dependencies*.

For instance, it is well known that drinkers can lose vitamin B1 very rapidly and thereby contract *Korsakoff's syndrome*. Mild cases can manifest as confusion and memory loss; not a great state for those who read and talk about the scriptures. In more severe cases, the *mammalary bodies* of the *hypothalamus* can hemorrhage, leading to a fast trip to the afterlife.

It less well known that the tremors associated with alcoholism may also be related to loss of *magnesium*, which works synergistically with vitamin C and the B vitamins.

The B vitamins are best given as a whole complex, including B1, B2, B3, B5, B6, and B12* etc, and may cause imbalances if given individually. For example, is has been common practice to provide B1 alone for *Korsakoff's syndrome*. This foolish practice can lead to physiological and therefore spiritual imbalance.

An appropriate amount of exercise can increase our metabolism, and help us absorb nutrients more efficiently, as one of the goals of the *human body design*. However, excessive practice of even good habits, like long distance running, aerobic exercise or sports, can diminish nutritional resources, causing imbalance.

The sense of well being associated with a runners or swimmers high is due to the production of *endorphins*. These *natural opiods* are produced by the body to presumably help mitigate the pain associated with fighting or fleeing from predators and are built into our genetic past.

---

*For those who have trouble absorbing certain B vitamins; b12, b1, etc – for a variety of reasons including lack of intrinsic factor – these vitamins are now available in high potency sublingual forms that melt on or next to the tongue.

When excessive exercise is happening, the body will produce not so good chemicals, including excessive cortisol. **

Note that some channels for the excitatory neurotransmitter *glutamate* are modulated by zinc and magnesium (95), which are necessary in the proper amounts to modulate the flow of the brain chemical. It is commonly known that the *omega 3 fatty acids*, including their vegetarian, mercury free, sources, can produce a sense of wellbeing, conducive to productive meditation practices. Proper amounts of *calcium, magnesium and zinc,* hopefully from readily absorbable - preferably food sources - are also necessary for the calm associated with spiritual practices.

The seizures of epileptics, the hallucinations of schizophrenics and the brain degeneration associated with Alzheimer's disease*, are all at least in part associated with excessive glutamate.

**Cortisol in excess can diminish immune function and produce a host of unwanted side effects, including compromised immune function.

* In many cultures, these are among the spiritual diseases often attributed to demons, curses or perhaps the evil eye.

Conversely, a sense of well being, associated with the production of certain feel *good neurotransmitters,* like serotonin (5HT), is also related to a balance of nutrients including carbohydrates, proteins, notable tryptophan, vitamins, including vitamin C. The B Vitamins, including pantothenic acid, niacin, folic acid, b1, b12,…are also mandatory for nervous system health.

The key to spiritual exercise is balance and moderation. Whether one is striving to do yoga or swimming, to release innate spiritual forces while releasing the feel good chemical, DHEA, or eating dark chocolate to increase antioxidants, while promoting feelings associated with love, through ingesting of phenylalanine, the key is moderation and:

BALANCE, BALANCE, BALANCE

Note that the relevance of spiritual medicine reaches far beyond the domain of the human organism and into the realm of the social system, including: the arts the humanities, the earth and perhaps the universe at large at some levels

Art and Health

Art has been used for clinical assessment as well as for therapeutic processes.

For example, in psychological assessment protocols, it is common to have a client draw physical structures, including, a house, a tree, a person, etc.

In these *well validated* and *reliable* tools, the shape and placement of windows, the expansiveness of the trees and facial expressions of the person drawn, are clues to the personality (long term characteristics) and moods (transient/short idiosyncrasies) of the person being drawn.

It may be important to *repeat* these tests in an attempt to differentiate between long and short term characteristics of the person under assessment.

From a therapeutic perspective, both the viewing of art and the creation of art have therapeutic consequences.

When viewing art there are deep seated mechanisms within the visual parts of the human nervous system that will respond to characteristic cues, found within nature and mimicked within art.

The viewing and appreciation of actual physical things in nature can have similar effects.

There are a variety of 'programs' built into the human visual system that help us to decipher relevant information from visual data.

For example, at a very basic level, *geons* (92) are used by the human nervous system to make sense out of basic shapes, like line, curves and sphere. They may be considered to be akin to building blocks which are used to construct more complex designs.

At another level of the brain, the *gestalt* concepts of symmetry (92) may goad humans to assume things that are simply not there.

For example, if three unconnected angles are placed at the vertices of an equilateral triangle, the visio-cognitive system will assume that the complete triangle is present.

The importance of symmetry is teleologically significant, in that the *healthy* human form is meant to be symmetrical. There is even evidence to suggest that a symmetrical human face is indicative of parenting capability (56).

Beautiful and healthy skin and nails and shiny hair are cues to potential mates, and to the world at large, that the person who possesses those attributes is a good candidate to help another healthy person pass on strong genes and thereby help the human race to survive.

Of course, in our complex technologically oriented, stress filled world, things may be going on genetically that are hidden at deeper levels (breaks, translocations, etc), so even beautiful humans may get sick these days.

Symmetry in nature may contain cues that remind us of the healthy humans that do indeed have symmetrical bodies that fit the proper ratio of *lip width to nose width*, skin and hair health themes, etc.

There are also many deeper and more subtle attributes of art that may also strike a cord with us at a variety of levels.

For example, these attributes may *remind us* of 'safe spaces where we may hide from ferocious predators from the distant past or conversely where we may readily obtain food.'

The *beauty* of these spaces may make us feel at *peace* or be *exhilarated* because they are *cues* to us that our *chances of survival are indeed good* and we have nothing to worry about.

Art can also be used to facilitate the creative aspect of the spiritual healing program.

Painting, sculpting, and crafts have been used for eons as a creative outlet for those suffering a variety of physical, emotional, or mental afflictions.

The wise clinician will 'let' creative folks do creative things. They are your customers, not the other way around.

Architecture and Sacred Spaces

I was once part for a team that was chartered with helping to make Yale New Haven hospital a more peaceful and customer oriented place for patients and their families. While the initial focus was on the reduction of unnecessary noise in patient areas, we seized the opportunity to apply *spiritual ergonomics*.

Our suggestions included all sorts of things from safe aromatherapy possibilities, some relaxing herbal teas for patients, and music carts filled with relaxing CDs to making waiting rooms in intensive care areas more pleasant for the families of those undergoing extreme trauma.

We all agreed that an aquarium might be a great stress reliever, since watching fish leisurely swim is a tried and true way to get anxious folks to relax.

We were also able to convince the powers that be that *relaxing murals*, especially with unique themes to guard against boredom in the different rooms, would be the way to go.

The use of a special color called *Baker-Miller Pink* has also been used extensively in hospital, jail and home settings to calm folks down.

Many years ago, I was the caretaker of a municipal building, while attending college at night. During that most interesting couple of years, I had the opportunity to change the lights in a police front desk area that was plagued with contributing to eyestrain and painting a holding cell to none other than Baker-Miller pink. Positive results manifested in both cases.

Emergency and surgery departments have also found that light blue colors have been successful in calming down patients in challenging situations.

Conversely, bright reds in those areas have been demonstrated to have the opposite affects.

There is lot of room for much needed research in these areas.

Of course, the spiritual healer is advised to learn about the healing environment in health care settings; including the strategic use of light, sound, color, *air ionization*, and even healing gardens and *labyrinths*, which are becoming popular today.

These human bodies that we inhabit have evolved over millions of years under natural conditions. It is now common knowledge that to live in harmony with our natural heritage that we must eat the right foods, exercise properly, and learn to manage our stress in a variety of ways. Many of us also know that it is important to be mindful of household environmental factors that may include radon, air borne molds, a variety of toxic waste products and some even heed the *Feng Shui* arrangement of our living spaces.

The ideal 'natural' living space would take into account the intensity, duration, and 'color' of the light. The optimal overall color are light sources that are close to natural sunlight or let sunlight in without blocking important parts of the light, including small amounts of the beneficial types of ultraviolet light. UV can help the eyes work properly and help to avoid eyestrain and associated headaches.

Air ionization is another important, yet often neglected factor in environmental design. Air ionization is the electrical charge of the air itself. Like the pole of a battery, air can be charged more positively or negatively. Negatively ionized air is partly responsible for the exhilaration we may feel at the seashore, in the mountains, and even in pine forests. Pine needles are said to emit negative electricity from the points of their needles. This electricity then charges the surrounding air. The 'point discharge' associated with pine needles may have something to do with the wonderful feelings we get while around Christmas trees and Chanukah bushes during that very special season. To enhance this effect in your living space, it may be important to use natural fibers and woods as opposed to plastics, vinyl, and synthetic carpeting which tend to attract the negative ions.

In earlier chapters, we introduced the human energy field. Now we will extend our discussion to include some relationships between the individual energy field and some relevant aspects of the environment. Many consider this relationship to be sacred in many ways.

Humans have evolved for countless eons under low level magnetic fields, natural sunlight, and pure clean air. As modern day humans, however, we are separated from our natural environment by our dwellings and workplaces. Even some types of synthetic clothing can have negative ramifications.

Polyester clothing, plastic furniture, and synthetic carpeting may carry what is called a positive electrical charge. This means that these synthetic materials can neutralize the healthy natural 'negative' charge in fresh clean air. This situation can lead to not only respiratory problems, but even some forms of depression. This is because negatively charged air has been linked to important chemicals in our brains, including serotonin, which are important to our sense of well being. Certain plants, including those with pointy needles, some types of splashing water fountains, and even negative ion generators have been helpful to some folk who are starved for negative ions. Natural fiber clothing, carpeting, and furniture can do wonders for those who are sensitive to ionization changes.

Man made electrical and magnetic systems may have adverse affects on our health. For instance, certain electrical appliances, including cell phones, electric blankets, and hair dryers are said to 'make matters worse' in susceptible individuals. Conversely, many claim that the use of magnets, cloths, bed and furniture coverings impregnated with magnetic fibers, and even magnetic insoles can do lots of good things for us. Relief from chronic pain, fatigue, and sleep disturbances are among the many benefits claimed.

We also know that humans thrive under light sources that simulate natural sunlight and that there is also an acceptable range of brightness.

In the 1960s, the nutrition (yes nutrition) department at MIT conducted a series of experiments in which rats were raised under two different lighting conditions.

One group of animals raised under light with high amounts of yellow color had what is called 'adrenal hyperplasia' (114). This means that their adrenal glands, which are important for stress management, were excessively large as though they had been under significant stress. Conversely, rats raised under light that was closer to the color of natural sunlight had normal adrenals. Similar experiments were repeated and verified by Japanese and American researchers (122). German researchers have found that stress chemicals tend to be higher in humans resting quietly under cool white lights than under full-spectrum light (121). Light that is too dim or too bright can also be stressful for humans. Many folks are now using full-spectrum lighting and/or full spectrum transmitting glass in their 'sacred spaces' for optimal well being *.

Most of all, it is important to realize that the human energy field interacts with light, air ionization, and magnetic fields at the same time. ~ so choose your sacred spaces well.

---

* Please note that the methods and procedures used in experiments presented in references sited are for information purposes and do not necessarily represent the views of the author.

Light and Health

The researcher who ignores the relevant environment is doomed to place often undetected confounds into their experiments. Conversely, the wisely constructed study, which is repeated over varying environmental *noise factors* (often uncontrolled conditions that may impact the experiment), will be a more reliable one.

Light can and does have a profound influence on the health and wellbeing of almost everyone and had best not be ignored.

Lighting is among the most important, yet least understood, environmental factor that can influence your health, vitality, strength, and even the quality and productivity of your work. Some studies have implied increases in productivity ranging from 0.5 to 5 percent by just changing the color of the light bulbs. The studies take into consideration factors besides the social factors found in the famous 'Hawthorne Study.' The physiological and psychological aspects of light itself can profoundly impact your ability to manage stress.

Throughout history, including in Egypt, India, Chine and elsewhere, healing systems have used light at very specific wavelength ranges (blue, red, yellow…) and intensities to heal very specific maladies. The specificity in terms of wavelength was often accomplished by passing light through colored glass, liquids, etc.

In more modern times, both high and low level lasers of exact frequencies and intensities have been used to stimulate energy meridians, burn and vaporize diseased tissue and even weld parts of the eye that have become detached.

The color and intensity of light is particularly important in health care settings (119), especially when people are most vulnerable to even the most subtle environmental influences

Light affects our health and performance in many important ways. It is well established that most people feel a sense of wellness on bright and sunny days and may feel 'under the weather' or even depressed, during long periods of light deprivation. In fact, the high winter suicide rates in Scandinavian countries, including Sweden, have long been attributed to lack of a very important 'nutrient' - *Light*.

It is well known that light is often used to treat the depression associated with *seasonal affective disorder*, commonly called SAD. These treatment affects are believed to be related to the breakdown of excessive melatonin in susceptible individuals. This breakdown of excessive melatonin, well know for its beneficial affects at healthy levels, has been attributed mostly to the amount of light received through the eyes.

When we think of light it is important to take into consideration both the intensity of the light and the color. Intensity is usually measured in lumens or *lux*. The color of light is typically measured in degrees Kelvin, as it is indirectly related to the light emitted from materials at specific temperatures. This measurement has to do with the proportions of different colors, which are combined to make up the light emitted from the source in question. As most of us know, when white light is passed through a prism, light of various colors emerge. The rainbow that appears in the sky after a rainstorm is based on similar principles.

While there is variation between the color and intensity of natural daylight, indoor lighting is often compared to sunlight. Most indoor lighting is much less intense than natural outdoor light, but the color of artificial lighting is often compared to sunlight. Light that is closest to natural sunlight is called full-spectrum light and is said to be about 90% true to natural daylight.

The more commonly used cool-white fluorescent lighting, is about 60% true to nature daylight and emits more yellow light than full spectrum light. This type of light is considered by many researchers to be more stressful than full spectrum light.

In fact, German researchers, Drs. Hollwich and Dieckhues, found that people sitting quietly under cool-white light tended to have higher levels of the stress hormones ACTH and cortisol than others under full-spectrum light (121). Others, including a team at MIT, found that rats raised under cool-white light or sodium vapor light had larger adrenal glands than those raised under full-spectrum light (114). Jacob Leiberman, Ph.D., OD has reported an interesting ramification to this research in his book, *Light: Medicine of the Future* (125). These findings indicate higher stress levels have led to administrators banning of cool-white light in several healthcare facilities throughout Germany.

Light has been used for millennia for the prevention and treatment of disease, and has been included in the ancient healing systems of India and Egypt. In more modern 'healing temples,' such as prenatal intensive care units, light is the treatment of choice for newborn jaundice.

Certain wavelengths in the bluish parts of the light spectrum are actually believed to break chemical bonds within the bilirubin molecule, which is associated with the breakdown of the mother's hemoglobin by the neonate's liver. Until recently, the conventional medical treatment for *hyperbilirumemia* was complete blood transfusion.

In more traditional cultures, new born babies are often put in the sun for short periods, for this reason; albeit it is doubtful that the parents would have a good idea of the etiology and morphology behind their babies yellow skin. In some cases the excess of bilirubin may lead to serious effects including death in some cases.

On the other hand, intense sunlight could be extremely damaging to the eyes and sensitive skin of newborns. The importance of multi cultural awareness can not be over emphasized here.

Light is also commonly used for the treatment of skin diseases such as psoriasis and may also be implicated in such diverse conditions as premenstrual syndrome and certain forms of arthritis. It is interesting that one of the first pioneers in modern light research, Dr. John Ott, had demonstrated significant improvements in rheumatoid arthritis after his sunglasses were broken. Ott concludes that the human visual system also has an endocrine function (123). The improvement was attributed to the fact that most conventional sunglasses will only allow certain parts of white light spectrum to pass through them, while blocking others.

Light may also impact our cognitive or thinking functions as well as having known relationships to the health of our bones and teeth. One of the earliest experiments related to full spectrum lighting was done in the Sarasota, Florida school system. It was found that *hyperactivity* in children was significantly reduced in classrooms where full spectrum light was used as opposed to other classrooms where conventional cool-white lighting was used.

Music and the Human Nervous System

The relationship between music and health has been a long and productive one. The healing power of harmony and beauty was well known in ancient civilizations, including Egyptian, Greek, Chinese, and Indian. Many ancient healing systems, including those promoted by Pythagoras, included music and color as important healing modalities.

In more modern times, conventional music therapy has been elevated to the level of neurology and neuroscience. Neuroscience is focused on research and academic study of the brain and nervous system. In this article we will touch upon some of the uses of music in healing and some of the proposed reasons why they work.

Dr. Connie Tomaino is a pioneer in music therapy and is a leader in 'Music and Neurology' at Beth Abraham hospital, where she works with the music therapist/neurologist, Oliver Saks. She is also an advisor for the CT Holistic Health Association. Dr. Tomaino's most inspiring talk a few years back at Yale included videos showing the benefits of music therapy in treating both Alzheimer's disease and Parkinson's disease. In the Alzheimer's case, an elderly patient who could barely mumble her words was actually able to sing songs after the treatment. In the Parkinson's case, an irregular gait was dramatically altered by the music therapy so that upon its completion, the patient's step had become regular and much smoother. It is believed that the rhythm of music may cause new connections to form within the brain that may in some way compensate for functions lost from these devastating diseases. The emotional impact of music may actually help to make these connections stronger and longer lasting.

Many universities, including Yale, UCONN, and Western Connecticut State University, are taking the 'music and the brain' concept very seriously.

Music has been commonly used as a relaxation agent for many years. More current innovations include CDs that mix soothing melodies with sounds designed to change brainwaves frequency and intensity. These methods typically include a series of clicking sounds that entice the brain to produce slower and more relaxing brainwave patterns. The clicking may be annoying to some people when listened to alone. However, when masked by Beethoven or healing sounds from nature, the beneficial effect may be twofold. The soothing music and the sound used to slow down the brainwaves may work together to produce an even more profound relaxation than either modality alone might. In some cases of depression, music has been used to *speed up* parts of the brain associated with depression. Conversely, in some cases of anxiety, regions of the brain have been *slowed down* by music based brainwave entrainment.

Don Campbell, author of *Music Physician for Times to Come*, tells us that music may have a powerful influence on the circulatory system. As early as the 1830s it was thought that "variations in circulation depend on pitch, intensity, and timbre of the sound". The possibilities in the control of some forms of hypertension are enormous.

The healing aspects of Gregorian chants, as well as the universal use of Eastern chants, including the 'sacred sounds' of *Hu* (60) and *Aum* are well known.

New innovations in the use of music therapy include its use to relax patients about to undergo surgery, dental work, and physical therapies

As I mentioned earlier, I once asked a panel of leaders at the Mayo clinic what they thought the medicine of the future might be like. One of the primary leaders thought that the direct uses of light, sound, music, and magnetic fields would play a key role in the future of medicine. Tone, rhythm, and harmony have clear and often time's powerful influences on prevention, wellness, and holistic healthcare.

Ethics and Spirituality

The is no place in society for unethical behavior and no place where unethical behavior may do more harm than in health care and in religious organizations. When patients lose their confidence in those that may help them, when they really need them, they tend to lose hope.

Unfortunately, these are among the very organizations that have experienced the most unethical behavior imaginable; including *in appropriate behaviors, rape, theft and tax evasion*. Problems with clinicians and students hanging around operating rooms for all the wrong reasons, including gawking at patients in various states of dress, are being seriously addressed, including dismissal and lawsuits in many hospitals.

Many organizations including surgery centers, are trying to playing it safe by automatically using same gender practitioners at every level, including talking therapeutics. Along similar lines, patient and clients dress codes are being reviewed and changed in many cases. For a variety of security concerns, security measures are being enhanced throughout the healthcare arena.

Some organizations are using cams to try to prevent problems. Unfortunately, in some of these very organizations, unethical practitioners and others, are using these very cams to spy on clients and patients in very inappropriate ways. As in locker rooms of all types, there have even been instances where inappropriate pictures have appeared on the internet at the expense of clients and patients.

The use of illegal and prescription drugs among the healing professions is also a very real danger to everyone.

On the positive side, patients and their families are more aware and savvy and have prosecuted many professionals for unethical behavior.

When I was a teen there was a very special area where lots of spiritual organizations would meet to discuss lots of very interesting ideas from their tradition.

Since I was much more interested in the *golden thread* through all religions, I would often play the *devil's advocate* by presenting opposing ideas to stimulate discussion.

For example, I would sometimes; discuss ideas from Eckankar with the born again Christians, Scientology with the Eckists, Jesus with the Hari Krishnas and so forth. There was also a high level church official that would chat with all the kids in the area, supposedly to help the kids stay safe and on track.

One nite, after a long round of religious banter, a high ranking Lutheran priest suggested that I come with him to the rectory to continue our discussion. As soon as I arrived he asked me if I wanted some drink and proceeded to give me some *communion wine!*

When I was about to leave, he said *that I shouldn't drive after drinking* and that I was welcome to spend the nite.

Just as I was about to go to sleep, I felt the approximately 6' 4," bodybuilder get in the bed next to me and tell me that, "anything is OK with God as long as there is love." When I kiddingly told him that I was not into what he was into, and that he should find me a cute nun instead, he got the hint.

That nite, I barricaded myself in the room by wedging a chair between the bed and the door amidst lots of guns, knives and barbells.

I learned a lot about *trust* and *breech of ethics* during that very scary nite, but did not appreciate the severity of the situation until many years later. As a teen, I thought it was quite funny, but as an adult I realized that I should have called my parents and the police to stop this predator in his tracks.

Since this incident did NOT involve a religion that has recently had much press about the subject; it was therefore proof that that sort of things was even more widespread than thought.

It is often said that just *because someone takes a course*, regardless of how difficult it may be, that it has little to do with their character, their morals, or with ethical behavior.

There are professional societies for most relevant professions that may keep records regarding misconduct in any of its myriad forms. Clinicians, researchers any/or educators, or clients, may want to educate themselves before they are involved with anyone who bring down their credibility or take advantage of them. Information from those who have worked with, or have been treated by, the 'spiritual practitioner' under scrutiny, may also provide potentially useful information.

In view of the many problems that are constantly being told in the press, those who are planning to bring someone into an organization, may also want to carefully check credentials, experience, and to have a release form in place so that any problems that may occur outside of the domain in question and not your legal responsibility, regardless of your perceived moral responsibility.

According to Anthony and Taylor (4), spirituality in the workplace may be defined succinctly as a set of seven principles, including: creativity, communication, respect, vision, partnership, flexibility and energy.

These and related principles may also be considered to be among viable ethical guidelines to consider for spirituality in healthcare.

One might consider categorizing these principles into two general levels. Those that allow and facilitate increased capability; including vision, flexibility, energy, and creativity, would tend to put the patient more in control of their own problem solving destiny.

When one feels a sense of self-control, they are naturally less stressed, more capable of healing themselves and therefore less liable of being depressed.

In situations where the patient really needs help or they perceive that they do, the 'spiritual principles' of communication, respect and partnership come into play.

From an ethical standpoint, those practices, policies and procedures that facilitate these principles, or a relevant subset, may be considered to be ethical in nature. On the other hand, when they suppress, block or discourage these concepts, without good reason, the survival potential of the patient is diminished. In those cases one might consider that the actions are unethical in nature.

For example, many patients are resourceful, intelligent, and capable these days. It is not uncommon for them in some cases to research and really know more that their caregiver about their plight.

Should a caregiver push a drug with significant side effects on a patient, or keep them coming for additional treatments that are not justified, to maintain their sense of power, control and/or profit, those actions would be considered to be unethical – even if the service was free of charge.

Besides, they would tend to also diminish the patient's sense of confidence, self-esteem and self-efficacy, if they were to become unduly dependant on others, including practitioners.

Caveat emptor – buyer beware

The Physician of the Future

There is no doubt in my mind that the successful physician of the future will be a *humanitarian*, with a bent towards holism and a dedication towards *'best practices'* from a broad array of possibilities. To be prepared for this daunting task, I believe that a very different emphasis will be required from pre-professional and professional education. This change needs to happen now.

We are in the midst of a paradigm shift in healthcare and wellness, not just in the United States, but throughout the world. The model has changed to a *patient-centric* one, focused upon prevention, therapeutic alliances, and holism. For most people, powerful drugs and surgery are last resorts. Instead, nutrition, stress management, and fitness are the hallmarks of the emerging model and patients are taking the lead in their own healthcare. In many parts of the US and indeed globally, there are areas where chiropractors are on every block and acupuncturists and naturopathic physicians are vying for office space in professional buildings. More women are going to women clinicians exclusively and both men and women are much more educated when it comes to healthcare. Self-care is also being practiced more often.

All of these considerations might be lumped into a broad category; one I have been very involved in, called 'holistic medicine.' Holistic medicine is a broad term, which implies the best practices, including, but not limited to, conventional and alternative medicine.

The hallmark of conventional medicine is the use of allopathic drugs and surgery, while the term alternative medicine implies the use of other practices to replace drugs and surgery. 'Complementary medicine,' on the other hand, implies a partnership between conventional medicine and alternative practices. The focus is on prevention, therapeutic alliances, patient centered approaches, and minimally invasive procedures. These might include minimally invasive surgery and non-pharmacologic approaches to pain management.

Alternative practices might encompass a variety of modalities, including, but not limited to traditional medicine (Chinese medicine, Tibetan medicine, Ayurveda, African Healing Systems, and Native American Healing), 'Energy' healing (Reiki, Therapeutic Touch, Healing Touch, and including a variety of distance healing and self healing modalities), bodywork, nutrition and/or chiropractic approaches. Another name for Complementary medicine is 'Integrative medicine.' This name was chosen to imply not only wholeness, but to fix a problem that the name complementary caused.

Patients thought 'complementary' implied that it was free!

Holistic medicine is the broadest relevant category and implies not only Alternative, Complementary and Integrative medicine, but much more. Holistic physicians (Including Allopathic, Homeopathic, Naturopathic, Osteopathic, and Podiatric) are only part of the story. Holistic nursing and dentistry are coming to the forefront. More esoteric practices, like body-mind psychotherapy, spirituality and health, organizational wellness, holistic architecture and landscaping and even CAM (complementary and alternative medicine) in neuroscience and humanities in medicine are making sweeping changes in the way we think about healthcare and wellness.

In some cases, ethical issues may be even more pronounced within the holistic community. Accordingly, many hands on approaches are being replaced with less potentially problematic hands off approaches.

There is no question in my mind that holistic healthcare is not only the wave of the future, but also the course of the present.

The primary goal of holistic organizations is to support holistically oriented practices while promoting partnerships with conventional medicine, academia, industry and government. These groups often sponsor conferences, symposia, professional health fairs and monthly networking educational meetings throughout the states where they are active.

My interest in holistic medicine goes back to my teen years in the 1970s when I had a stubborn bout with pneumonia. I tried conventional medicine, including antibiotics and sulfa drugs, for nearly a year with no success. Both physicians I worked with were at a loss as to how to treat me and the drugs were making me feel awful. Finally, being the rebellious teen that I was, I decided to take matters into my own hands. In just three weeks of using self-applied nutritional approaches, my pneumonia was completely gone and it has never returned. My treatment included minimizing dairy products, eating more fresh fruits and vegetables and taking some vitamin supplements. No one bothered to ask me about my diet. If they had they might have realized that, like many teenage boys of the time, I was into a high-protein diet full of dairy and lacking in fresh veggies (against my parents wishes) and vitamins. Many others are taking healthcare into their own hands.

There are hundreds of internet sites relating to health and interested consumers visit wellness and these sites millions of times per month. In fact, many of the physicians I know have commented that due to their busy schedules that they often can not keep up with their patients in terms of current information.

My interests in psychology, neuroscience, and electrical engineering gave me a strong appreciation for ways where all of these areas would eventually merge for the betterment of humanity. Interests in East/West spirituality also made me mindful of the many ramifications concerning what we might tap into. This composite view made me mindful of both huge potential mixed with huge responsibility.

Strides in 'electro-medicine' including imaging and non-invasive blood testing are only part of the emerging story. Chiropractors now use thermal detectors to assess problems with spinal alignment. Electro-acupuncture has the potential to preserve the best of traditional Chinese medicine while providing new non-invasive ways to deal with not only pain, but also a litany of medical problems. Lasers are rapidly becoming the hallmark of many *minimally invasive* surgical and dental procedures and the huge potential for low-level lasers is virtually untapped. Hands off and distance healing processes are also being taken more seriously as medical innovations.

One aspect of innovation at the *Mayo Clinic* was the team-based approach pioneered by the Mayo brothers at the turn of the last century. Another aspect involves *electro-medicine*. They suggested that light, sound, electricity and magnetic fields would play a major role in prevention and diagnosis. There were also implications that in the future the need for physicians might eventually go away entirely.

Researchers also know that ambient lighting, color, sound, music, air ionization and even art and architecture may have significant ramifications on the health of human system.

Some physicians also realize that *spirituality* can be most important to patients and that *multi-cultural diversity* may add significant complexity to case management.

In view of these emerging trends, the physician of the future may play a very different role than the typical physicians of today. The emerging model will be different from a variety of perspectives. In fact, the rapidly emerging healthcare and wellness model is clearly a broad-based bio/psycho/social/techno/spiritual one with many roots and cultural ramifications.

Patients themselves are mostly interested in preventing illness and getting well rapidly with minimal cost. Driven by both *intrinsic motivators* and *societal pressures*, physicians of many persuasions, including allopathic, osteopathic, naturopathic, chiropractic, and oriental medicine, while having their differences, are working together to provide total solutions. It is now common for medical and osteopathic students to study alternative and complementary approaches, while students of chiropractic and naturopathic healthcare are most interested in learning about relevant drug and surgical approaches.

It is most likely that progressive universities will have common pre-clinical programs where future MD's, ND's, DO's, DC's, and OMD's will take their first two years together, before branching off into their special fields. Further evolution will most likely lead to interdisciplinary programs, such as MD/ND, DO/OMD, MD/PsyD and a variety of special certificates en route to their physician degree. Nutrition, stress management, pain management acupuncture will most likely be among the mix of many current certificate options. Future certificate programs will more likely involve more hands off and distance healing options. Even more comprehensive composite degree programs of a holistic nature are on the horizon. Perhaps these interdisciplinary programs may be called *master physician programs*. In any event, new degree innovations are likely to have a stronger emphasis on prevention and patient education, with a focus on stress management, patient responsibility and customer satisfaction.

Excessive stress accounts far more than 50% of all medical visits and excessive stress due *to intrinsic and extrinsic conflict* is among the most prevalent and insidious banes of modern organizations. The responsible physician of the future will certainly need to know more about organizational dynamics of the workplace if she/he wants to successfully understand their patients' disease processes and how to help them. Individual differences and patient respect will also take precedence. The practitioner must eventually realize that even the presence of the 'wrong' practitioner, in terms of gender, approach, manner, religious conviction, etc....does have profound influence on the therapeutic process. In fact, the wrong practitioner from form the *patient's perception*, can do more harm than anything therapeutic that they may have to offer.

While professional curricular innovations are already happening, there is also much room for pragmatic innovation in the pre-professional curriculum. Given the high demands of future professional education, what better place than pre-professional education to set the stage, all the while making optimal use of overall educational time? My training as an engineer has encouraged me towards efficient and effective innovation.

With these technological innovations already emerging, the need for memorization in subjects like organic chemistry and physics may have much less value for the future physician. With innovations like the internet, one may capture the most up to date information with a few keystrokes.

More efficient and effective use of pre-professional educational might include case-based subjects which will best prepare future physicians, nurses, dentists and others for the future. Emerging courses might have names like *holistic wellness and healthcare excellence*, *anthropological views of traditional healing*, *organizational behavior and stress*, *spirituality and health*, *multi-cultural diversity*, and *humanities, the arts and health*, and, *nutrition and fitness in the workplace*. A variety of pre-professional certificates may be of considerable benefit to motivate students along these proposed pre-professional tracks. *Professional ethics* is a must.

Remember it's *not* about you, your students, residents, interns or anybody else but the customer and their needs.

The Spiritual Organization of the Future

The ideas and innovations conveyed in *Spiritual Medicine* would be much easier to implement if grounded in a supportive organizational structure, including, but not limited to the university.

The university system has always been an important part of many readers' lives and I have learned that several of you have contemplated what the *University of the Future* might be like. In my estimation, this idyllic 'system of systems' would be based upon both holism and humanitarian constructs within the framework of significant social relevance and 'optimal survival.' By the way, the same set of tenets might also apply to religious systems if you think carefully about it.

The term 'optimal survival' is used here to imply that courses and curricular programs would be designed such that graduates could readily apply the principles learned in ways that would help improve the lives of themselves, their families, their places of employment, and society in general. The model proposed would be especially relevant for universities with professional schools. The systems based approaches proposed were designed to build a strong education foundations that would prepare graduates to enter the especially innovative and broad-based professional programs proposed.

Along with many other people who live in Southwestern Connecticut, 9/11 was a wake up call to me (Michael) regarding how finite and precious life is. This event was important in helping me to focus this idea while I'm still here! At the suggestion of friends and colleagues, I decided to turn these ideas into a 'virtual university' by creating a website, which I decided to call TCAM or *Total Complementary and Alternative Medicine, although the concept reaches far beyond the domain the TCAM.*

While the idea spans an entire university or perhaps a consortium of universities, the initial TCAM model has *a* focal point in healthcare and leadership. However, the scope of the 'TCAM model' is much broader and far reaching in scope and intention. The overriding theme would be a truly integrative model based upon *interdisciplinary cooperation, collaboration, and social relevance*. In my view, this futuristic system would purposefully facilitate responsible *analysis* in combination with broad-based *synthesis*. This systems construct could be exemplified in a variety of ways, including socially relevant projects that span large sectors of one university, or a consortium of schools, government, and business enterprises.

For example, a favorite projected project for the TCAM based university would be the development of the 'ideal' healthcare systems. As a collaborative effort, humanistically oriented constructs from

Architecture, forestry (landscaping), art, music and the humanities, could supply a structural framework for the process of holistically oriented healthcare to emerge, develop and grow in systemic and organized ways. The proposed *healthcare provider of the future* would be allowed to thrive in this ideal environment, but from the spiritual perspective, would be strongly encouraged to contemplate the Hippocratic Oath from a much broader bio/psycho/social purview and little room *for unethical and/or self centered* behavior.

The more spiritual healthcare organization would be *patient centered*, with due and carefully consideration for the important details within the bigger system. Everything from *food options*, how *patients are expected to dress*, *who is allowed to observe procedures*… would be controlled by the patient and strictly enforced by the 'workers;' not the other way around.

As 'co-creators' of these constantly evolving and *continuously improving* systems, engineers, architects, nurses, physician associates, psychologists, and a variety of other holistically oriented health professionals would be encouraged to reach their full potential as not only healers, but as *respectful and patient oriented* teachers. The subjects taught would of course place a heavy emphasis on *nutrition, fitness and stress leadership*. Teachers would also openly communicate ways to teach patients to help themselves in many ways.

As preparation for this role, significant curricular innovations would not only be encouraged, but designed in efficient and effective ways inclusive of basic, clinical, and post graduate levels. For instance, nutritional and stress related constructs are easily meshed into courses like biochemistry, physiology, and neuroscience. Anatomy and pathology might be great places to better understand and include constructs from traditional and popular healthcare. Like it or not, constructs like the *acupuncture meridian* and the *chiropractic 'subluxation'* are common knowledge among patients and are here to stay. I think that the healthcare professional of the future would gain much by understanding the pros and cons of such approaches. Otherwise, their future patients may learn about them first!

I think that a clear and broad understanding of *multicultural diversity*, *organizational dynamics*, *quality systems*, and *business leadership* will be particularly important as mandatory aspects of clinical and post- graduate curricular innovation. Non-pharmacologic approaches to pain management will not only save countless lives potentially lost to 'iatrogenic' illness, but I believe that even the drug companies will invest in such approaches. Some of them are already interested in botanicals, nutrasuticals and even such unlikely innovations as 'music therapy' and Chinese medicine. The TCAM model provides for interdisciplinary and interdepartmental collaboration and cooperation within all of these arenas. Many broad-based programs and projects are envisioned as joint ventures between schools of *management*, *medicine*, *music*, *art*, and *divinity*.

The introduction of *humanistic and holistic* constructs into existing interdisciplinary programs, such as neuroscience, will bring dramatic innovations into our understanding and management of stress, strain and associated pathophysiology. By expanding such proposed innovations into collaborations with business management and leadership, the potential for the prevention and alleviation of human suffering is astronomical. Such enormously relevant Public Health innovations would easily save 100's of billions of dollars in stress related illness within the US alone. In this regard, TCAM based educational models, within neuroscience and business areas alone would *prevent untold waste* in terms of absenteeism, insurance claims, and violence in the workplace. These are all areas of understanding that the business leader, physician, PA, and nurse of the future would benefit greatly from and should be a mandatory part of curricular designs. What more important health concepts are there than understanding and managing stress within the workplace and school systems? Of course, nutrition (including obesity control) and fitness are also extremely important for both business leadership and healthcare.

The TCAM model could readily be applied to such potentially important 'curricular clusters' as certificate programs in *holistic leadership*, *music, art and wellness*, and *spirituality and health*. From another angle, interdisciplinary clusters in architecture, engineering, biophysics, and forestry can bring about living and healing spaces that are very efficient and highly effective in facilitation optimal health. Such considerations as the color and intensity of light, the ionization and oxygen levels of air, and optimal uses of color, art and sound, are no longer esoteric concepts, but are rapidly emerging towards the forefront of human understanding and wisdom.

Of course, anthropology, philosophy, literature, and other aspects of the humanities are no longer considered by many as 'necessary evils' of liberal arts education. I think that these are areas of considerable social relevance and are at least as important as the hard sciences are in pre-professional and professional education.

At first glance, the *system of systems* model I have proposed may seem daunting and especially impossible for those whose efforts are naturally focused upon the minutest of details. Within the proposed TCAM model, there are a variety of places where the details of the proposed curricular innovation would need to be developed and implemented. There would also be a need for the application of broad-based systems approaches that would naturally fall into the arenas of educational leadership.

I think that a steering committee comprised of *leadership leaders* applying TCAM principles would naturally include 'core team' leaders from schools of *healthcare*, *management*, *education*, *art*, *architecture*, and *divinity*. The structure, function, and scope of this proposed committee, would be dependant upon the university (or system of universities) implementing the innovation.

I have included an ongoing 'virtual draft' of the TCAM innovation. Of course, the name is arbitrary and the model itself is based upon its own principles, including continuous expansion and improvement.

TCAM site:
http://home.netcom.com/~mb1234/tcam1.0_001.htm

Divine Love

One might consider that *human love* is what makes the human race 'go round.' It is based upon *survival* of the individual, the family and the race itself.

Even the love for and by our pets, which can be among the best healers, is a love based on *symbiotic survival strategies*. Nothing mystical or complicated about any of this stuff.

I once had a gut feeling that I should go outside *asap* or there was going be trouble somewhere. Many of you know that strong gut feeling that you can not resist. *Intuition* at it's finest.

In an instant, a large turkey vulture swooped down and caught a snake in its strong beak.

Within minutes, a little abandoned squirrel wobbled out of its nest and made its way down it's tree as its life depended upon it. It did! It seemed as though it somehow knew what was going at the far end of the yard. Danger was there and it sure was.

That little babe followed me so intently that I was concerned at bit until I realized what was going on. It's mom had left it alone as I then surmised from the cries heard for almost a week, that it was starving.

The little creature had no fear of me whatsoever. In fact, it curled up on my shoe to keep warm and safe I assume; then it proceeded to climb up my leg for food and drink.

Fed it some nuts, but also learned that you can't give a baby squirrel water unless you know what you are doing, even if you think it might be dehydrated. I did think that and it turned out that I was somehow correct, according to the wild animal specialist we were able to find through a local nature center.

I loved that little squirrel, and did not want it to go, but thought it was best that I did. It was the cutest little animal I had ever seen and since we humans have a deep connection to cuteness that may have had something to do with it; even though it was a different species than my own.

People seek a mate that at both conscious and unconscious levels gives us the best chance to *survive teleologically at a variety of levels*.

We are more apt to spread our genes with a mate that we perceive as being *healthy** *a*nd *capable* as verified through:

---

*Note that in complex societies, and over eons of time, deep seated genetic abnormalities may still be present within the genetic code of a physically beautiful person.

1) A beautiful face, with consideration for healthy skin, symmetry, divine ratios (such as the width of the lips to the width of the nose) & cultural idiosyncrasies.

2) A well proportioned body

3) Characteristic voice which is high for females and deep for males

Once *our requirements* are met: including, personality, interests, hobbies, perceived fidelity.... there is a circuit in the brain that *switches on* and starts the human *love process*, with the sometimes hidden goal of providing healthy bodies for *body factory Earth*.

While absence sometimes makes the heart grow fonder, there is another circuit in the brain that tends to make us feel more connected to those that we *may see more often*. Perhaps a switch is turned on after a counter *counts a number of encounters* that make the object of our relationship more familiar.

This same circuit makes us feel connected to our families, which if things are OK, we naturally feel a strong sense of love for; mom, dad, sis, brother, and even Fido.

After all, there is protection in numbers and those beings that we tend to be around often, if they do not contribute to hurting us, may be perceived as helping us and therefore *enhancing our survival potential*. Our love for them is in reality our perception that will aid the survival of our offspring in some innate way.

We are more apt to *forgive* those whom we love also for some very good survival benefits. When someone hurts us, there are built in mechanisms associated with *fight or flight response,* thru the sympathetic part of the autonomic nervous system and the HPA axis, which put us in a state of alertness. This tense state is associated with perceived danger, even at deep unconscious levels. *When we forgive someone we are at some level turning off the switch associated with the danger response.*

Forgiveness also has something to do with *accepting things we can not change*, including but going beyond personal relationships to even *forgiveness of oneself.* These different forms of acceptance may also mean that we are turning off the *having to pay attention to a very dangerous situation 'switch'* and redirecting our energy to the tasks at hand. Forgiveness and acceptance are forms of loving ourselves by releasing unnecessary tension.

By *doing unto others ethically and responsibly* we are helping to create a better planet in which to live in, while avoiding reactive physiological processes that make us always be on guard for danger. After all, when we hurt, it is expected that we will be hurt back at deep levels of the brain.

Some folks at some very deep and even unconscious levels may want some anti-survival things, including inappropriate substances and other ways to fulfill their self destructive tendencies. We best be on guard regarding those who may take advantage of us to avoid *learning lessons the hard way*.

Even by *giving space and freedom to others*, especially our young children and other beings whom we may be in a place to guide, we are helping the planet grow as God wants – as long as we act responsibility, with appropriate intentions, while acting with due diligence.

I once had a friend that decided he would show his love to his puppy, by giving it as much space as possible and not encroaching on its fun. Unfortunately, *with freedom comes responsibility*, and this very irresponsible little puppy had a short life and a painful ending under the wheels of an irresponsible driver.

In affect, *the love we get is in some way really equal to the love we give and in the end truly meant for us*, like the song goes. At least at some very deep levels.

When we are *grateful* for the things we have in this world, we tend to remove our focus upon the *cognitive dissonance* or disconnect between that which we want and that we can't readily have, and therefore feel more at peace and once again are also helping ourselves.

Several years ago, I was interested in what someone had to say about *the ascension*. Coincidentally, I picked up some information on the subject in Connecticut, and tried to contact the person who wrote the materials and who just happened to live in California. She never returned my call, and I was on to other things, forgetting about my interest in the subject.

Six months later, and through a series of changes at work, I found myself in California on a work assignment, when I worked for a fortune 500 company. One evening I was out in a wooded area and got this inner prompting to ask a couple near by if they knew this person I tried to contact six months prior in Connecticut.

The woman swiftly replied that 'they have been waiting for me' and lots more. At first I was a bit skeptical until she proceeded to tell me lots about my life that no mere stranger could possibly know. Then she proceeded to tell me that I would be leading a very interesting group; but that I was not even close to ready to lead it and that it would take me about ten years before my training would bring me to the point of being an appropriate leader. I was told that I would be involved in the deepest of both academic and popular topics that were relevant to my 'project.' The projection was very true indeed.

One day I met a *student of chi* at a seminar at the Mayo Clinic on medical imaging. Get the picture? After a little more than ten years filled with similar relevant experiences, coincidences, you name it, I was asked to take the lead of a very interesting organization. Just like she said, about ten years!

By now it should be clear that the way that we study, teach or practice spiritual medicine has little to do with an inflexible template and lots to do with the viewpoint, sometimes changing, of the relevant student, population or client at hand. We not only have to consider multicultural diversity to be effective. *Higher power diversity* must be considered. The spiritual clinician, educator and researcher who has read this little book will have a better understanding of diversity at a variety of levels and depths within each level. That being said, even the level of the higher power itself is open to a diverse understanding among a variety of spiritual adherents. For example, there are many religions that believe that God is a male and that *He* at a level somewhere between the *astral* and the mental planes of existence.

Still other groups conclude that *the real God* resides at a level beyond the planes of matter, energy, space and time as we know them, and that God is neither male nor female. At yet another level of gradation, it is concluded that real real God resides several levels beyond the first manifestation of the divine being, just beyond the material worlds.

It also appears that where we put our interests also has something to do with where the higher power manifests in our lives. If we resonate with the *material aspects of the higher power* the focus will be on manifesting excellence in the here and now. However, if our focus is on the *more spiritual aspects of the higher power* our interests might be more involved with which *heaven* to reside in an the afterlife - or which ones to visit while still maintaining a physical body on Earth if we have those capabilities as some religions claim.

After all is said and done, the love for the *spirito-material multiverse* (112) may take precedence over everything else as we naturally *be* what is in the best interest of all that is and 'ever can be, in all the universes that *ever were* and ever *are possible*,' for the fun of it.

We may also seek guidance from other humans along the way.

~

Pastoral Counseling

Many patients consider the healing system to be a composite one, with their spiritual or religious system or systems of choice as very important parts thereof. Many also consider that their spiritual advisors can be the most successful aspect of their healing and/or grieving process.

Unfortunately, many spiritual advisors may be ill equipped to deal with complicated psychological issues that may be a huge part of the person's illness.

Counselors are trained to help people to cope with tough issues in life, and may often refer the patient to others with a more in depth clinical background, such as clinical psychologists and/or physicians, social workers, occupational therapists, etc. They may also work with other family members or significant others in the workplace to better understand psychological and social factors important to the case.

Research projects related to ascertaining the efficacy of counseling programs must by necessity be holistic in nature and take into consideration the holistic, bio.psycho.social, systems approach or they are doomed to fail.

For example, the nurse/counselor who neglects to consider the *dynamics of the workplace* where the patient works, and her impending termination in a recession economy, may have no clue why the patient no longer has any faith *in a higher power has lost hope* and *may be suicidal.*

According to Hunter (49), "What distinguishes pastoral counseling from other forms of counseling and psychotherapy is the role and accountability of the counselor and his or her understanding and expression of the pastoral relationship. Pastoral counselors are representatives of the central images of life and it's meaning affirmed by their religious communities. Thus pastoral counseling offers a relationship to that understanding of life and faith. Pastoral counseling uses both psychological and theological resources to deepen its understanding of the pastoral relationship."

So then, pastoral counselors integrate relevant aspects of psychology and/or psychiatry, with the core concepts of the religion that they are affliated with.

A pastoral counselor from the Jewish faith might takes core ideas from the Torah, such as *moral codes*, and carefully integrate these themes with moral concepts, and other ideas, from clinical and couseling psychology.

For example, a young man who constantly breaks the *ten commandments* might conceivably be asked to read the scriptures carefully and come to the synagouge more frequently, along with more conventional psychotherapeutic processes.

However, the devient person under scruteny may simutaneously be considered to be the worst type of anti-social personality type, the psychopath.

The responsible pastoral counselor may also consider that psychopaths are often *dangerous and hurtful to others*, and that they are *infrequently rehabilitated satisfactorily*.

Under these circumstances, and as act of *divine love* for others in the congregation, the pastoral counselor could conceivably find that he is a great danger and might find ways to isolate the young man from others for the safety of others in his flock. While there may be other therapeutic processes possible…., things that are done for the highest good of many, and done in a reasonable amount of time, may be the most appropriate approach.

Since pastoral counselors may have a signifigant understanding about the family circumtances in their congregation, they may be among the most likely people to help get to the real crux of the problems, many of which are environmenal in nature.

For example, the girl who has been raped or the guy who lives with a woman who constantly lies or shop lifts on a regular basis, may not get rid of their stomach upsets no matter what may be done for them in therapy.

First and formost, the spritual healer needs to know the environmental circumstances surrounding their patients lives.

The astute clinician will also look for signs of lying. For instance, the patient who has a source of anxiety in the form of a live-in drug addict, may not even come close to telling you why she is so tense all the time or where her money is really going.

Whe someone is telling the truth, their facial expressions will often be confirmation. Truthful people, for instance, will smile from the jaw area and the eye areas simultaneously. The *zymaticus* muscles in the lower ckeek will contract along with the *obicularus occuli* muscles surrounding the eyes.

In those who lie, only the lower cheek muscles will contract when they smile.

There is also a region above the bridge of the nose that will contract when someone lies. While this contraction is for only a fraction of a second, and requires very sophisticated equipment for detection, the CIA caught a US president by filming him and using time lapsed photography.

The lier may in some cases look towards the right when they are lying, presumable duw to it's conneciton with the *right creative side* of the brain.

The lying patient may also change their voice tones in characteristic ways and exagerate parts of stories that they are trying to hide, counterintuitive as that may seem.

The asute spiritual clinician/counselor will research the *lying literature*, etc, very carefully if they really want to help their patients, understand their research and even know what their students are really up to.

Perhaps the most powerful environmental stressor of them all is the *death or impending death* of someone close to them.

The wise spiritual researcher might also consider this most powerful, and often overlooked, potential confound.

Epilogue

As living beings on this most intriguing planet, the concept of death is perhaps the most interesting adventure of them all. If we think about the Hindu trilogy, we can view this most powerful concept as a fact of nature in these lower worlds of creation. The concept of *Vishnu the creator, Krishna and sustainer and Shiva the destroyer* also have counterparts in Western biomedicine.

During the period of biological development, we can now readily understand the union of the sperm and egg and how the fertilized ovum is programmed to develop into an embryo, fetus and eventually a fully functioning human being.

As the human progresses into childhood, adolescence and adulthood, a healthy being will naturally seek *high survival nourishment*. Of course, we can be fooled, as the sweets that some among us crave may in some ways are a dangerous substitute for mother's milk. The drive for survival will also lead humans to seek parental nurturing, interesting and creative employment, to seek beautiful and healthy mates and to spread our genes towards the continuous survival of the race.

But what about when the cellular system starts to degenerate? Does the being naturally seek death, first piecemeal through programmed cellular mechanisms, then through organ system dissolution and then eventually through the leaving of the physical body.

Then what?

Is it the role of the healer to keep the human being in it's decaying shell?

Perhaps there is value to such practices. But then again, is it also viable that we as spiritual beings are using these human frames as learning tools; learning the rules of nature and human experience so that we may eventually become experienced co-creators of the universe. Lots of folks believe these ideas, while still others consider these ideas to be the domain of heretics or perhaps lunatics or even worse, magicians.

What about reincarnation and past life recall? Some believe that these are just biological mechanisms in which genetic material is passed along through our genetic ancestry. Others believe that we are spiritual beings who take our experiences along with us from life to life. Then, still others believe that we are *both genetic and spiritual beings* who can remember both our genetic as well as our spiritual past.

From the spiritual perspective, do we then have spiritual goals geared towards *spiritual survival*? If so, then do heroic medical efforts to keep the dying in these bodies lay contra to the survival of our 'spiritual bodies?'

Many of our eastern brothers and sisters do believe that there are many planes of existence, and even life on these different levels. Called by many names, eastern and westerners alike might believe that there is an *astral plane*, then one where our karma or cause and effect 'bodies' reside. Some call this plane the *causal plane*, which is followed by planes leading up to the *unconscious plane* and then to even planes where there are *purely spiritual beings*.

Sound far fetched? Maybe so, but many religious traditions have some such schema, complete with some semblance of heaven and hell, cause and effect and differing views on death.

The next frontier in spiritual medicine is not the brain and nervous system, but perhaps what is far beyond all that and maybe beyond matter energy space and time all together.

Happy pondering as mere speculation evolves into deeper and more profound understanding of things above and beyond.

~ As Above, so Below. As Within, so Without ~

HU

~ and that which is beyond even that which is and that which is not and even beyond the light that was and is, and the word of God, and the great silence and that which is beyond even that~

~The Beginning~

Notes by you and for you

Notes by you and for you

Appendix I

13 Step program for spiritual well being

The following steps have been taken from the companion guide entitled

"The 13th
Step: the secret to becoming a coworker with the higher power of GOD"

13 Step program for spiritual well being

1) Educate ourselves about ourselves, our world and the world of spirit
2) Practice proper nutrition first and foremost
3) Integrate proper exercise and rest into our lives
4) Live effectively in the present, including meditation and contemplation in our daily lives
5) Take responsibility for our actions and inactions and take action in a timely fashion
6) Seek the help of others carefully if and when we really need it
7) Communicate relevant ideas clearly, concisely and appropriately & respect the awesome power of prayer and use it appropriately
8) Learn to listen carefully to relevant others
9) Live ethically within the laws of our society and avoid and ignore those who ignore them
10) Plan strategically for the future with due consideration for past history
11) Be considerate of others and do unto them ethically but without being taken advantage of
12) Listen carefully to the voice of the higher power through intuition, serendipity, coincidence & dreams

13) If you choose and you are asked in some way, consider becoming a coworker with the higher power of spirit under the direction of God and have fun doing so

Appendix II

Abbreviated experimental protocol for suggested studies on traumatic grief

While this section on innovation regarding TG is meant for the researcher, the astute clinician and educator can readily apply core concepts to their respective areas, which might include assessment, intervention, and cost related strategies and tactics, in related areas or perhaps different ones entirely.

Of course, in all cases, the spiritual professional is expected to apply these ideas in the most *ethical and customer centric* ways. Remember, 'it's not about you!"

Assessment Plan: In the first proposed experiment a sample of TG syndrome suffers, as confirmed by the Traumatic Grief Evaluation of Response to Loss Scale (Prigerson et al 2000), will be compared with a sample of those suffering from major depression without complicated bereavement and an aged matched control group. Comparisons to PTSD and OCD, both without complicated bereavement, are also being considered. All groups might be assessed initially for tendencies towards depression and suicide. These measures would be used as a screen for the control group. Smoking, alcohol and weight profiles could be conducted for each group. Cardiovascular, endocrine and immunological correlates may also be assessed for each group. An intervention strategy, which includes exercise and structured relaxation as described in the next section, could then be implemented across all groups.

After a period of three months, all assessments might be repeated, including the TRG2L in the confirmed TG syndrome group. Intergroup comparisons could be made as well as a comparison between the confirmed TG group and national statistics. The decision to use national statistics outside of the experimental cohort, in lieu of an additional non-treated control group, could be made so that interventions would not be withheld in a population with such a high risk for mortality and morbidity. The potential assessments could be repeated again at six months and then at nine months and one year. At the one-year assessment a detailed illness profile would also be added to the other assessment criteria.

Note that peak nocturnal melatonin levels would be measured in those patients with insomnia lasting more that 3 mo.

Intervention Strategy: The initial intervention strategy would be behavioral in nature and consist of co developing and implementing exercise and relaxation plans with the sample groups. Participative management has long been used to facilitate buy-in and the adherence to objectives in a variety of settings. In this context, the use of participation has the potential additional benefit of enhancing feelings of *self-efficacy*. The manifold benefits associated with actual participation in the exercise/relaxation program include enhanced feelings of self-esteem associated with improved body image and self-efficacy associated with a sense of accomplishment. The opportunity also exists for the TG sufferer to be encouraged to exercise in groups with other TG patients or those not suffering from the syndrome. The combination of enhancements in *self-esteem* and self-efficacy, along with possibly working with others, may greatly improve social functioning. There would also be expected improvements from *negative life-style behaviors* inherent in the TG syndrome. There are several direct biological benefits expected from both exercise and relaxation.

Direct cardiovascular benefits include improvements in lipid balance, such as the elevation in high-density lipoproteins and associated HDL: LDL ratio. This is an important consideration regarding arterioscleroses and total vascular resistance. Increases in *after load vascular resistance* are directly related to primary hypertension and cardiac hypertrophy. Secondary responses to arteriosclerosis include endocrine mediated elevations in blood pressure through the renal *renin-angiotensin* system. Improvements in cardiac efficiency are well known to be associated with exercise. Indirect cardiovascular benefits include improvements in catechlamines and glucocorticoids regulation after an adaptation period. Stress hormones enhance endorphin release through the hypothalamus and subsequently down regulates their release through a regulatory feedback loop. Importantly, Maslov et al (1999) has demonstrated that agonists of the *mu opiod receptor* increase the resistance of the heart to epinephrine, certain types of arrhythmias and ventricular fibrillation. As described in detail in the section on alcoholism, endorphins may also play a key role in preventing or reversing alcohol abuse so common in the TG population.

After signing an *informed consent form*, and being given written permission by their primary provider or approved designate, each participant would be given a choice of three exercise modalities, which are to be performed at least three times per week and which include:

- Walking at least one mile
- Swimming at least 1/4 mile
- Aerobics for 20 minutes

The participant will keep a *standard log* of their exercises, which will be given to then. The participant could bring this log to each three-month assessment. A member of the experimental team would randomly call participants on a biweekly basis to assure conformance and to facilitate ongoing communication and socialization.

Structured relaxation exercises are well known to facilitate adaptation to stress and to mediate the regulation of catechlamines and glucocorticoids. The benefits include improvements in immune response. Antoni et al (2000) assessed urinary cortisol levels in study involving 47 men who were given structured relaxation techniques. *Post-treatment effects, as compared to controls, include significant reductions in urinary cortisol and were correlated with improvements in self-reported measures of affect, anxiety, anger and confusion.* Crues et al (2000) found decreases in blood cortisol in breast cancer patients who practiced a cognitive-behavioral stress management regime. The same group, Crues et al (2000), found significant decreases in salivary cortisol in response to home relaxation practice in another study involving 30 gay men. McGrady et al (1991) found significant *decreases in blood glucose* in diabetics, between pre and post treatment measures, after following a 10-week biofeedback-assisted relaxation program. Rosenbaum (1983) had similar findings in another biofeedback study involving diabetics. All of these findings are important in the TG patient who is particularly prone to stress induced dysfunction in both mood and physiology; including the potential for blood sugar dysfunction.

Each participant might again be given a choice of modalities for structured relaxation. The relaxation sessions would be performed 5 times per week and would be logged by the participant. They include:
➢ Listening to one of three relaxation tapes which would be provided. The patient would be given three tapes to *avoid monotony* while providing the opportunity for making their own choice.
➢ Standard meditation protocols, such as TM (117).

> Join a relaxation class involving a *cognitive-behavioral* stress reduction program. An approved list would be provided to the participant. (in-house development or collaboration may be considered)

A tuition grant of up to $100 might be provided to each participant who chooses to take a relaxation course or class.

Hypothetical cost of assessment and intervention:

Preliminary estimates [per participant]

Psychometrics:
- Assessment - Four times at 1 hr per assessment
- Analysis - Four times at 0.5 hrs per assessment

Physical assessments (Optional):
- Electrocardiogram and assessment
- Lab work for endocrine assessments
- Lab work for immunological study

Interventions:
- Orientation session
- Phone audits of conformance
- Tapes
- Outside class or course [up to $100]

Feasibility assessments
- Initial assessments and interventions
- Further assessments and interventions

References and Suggested Readings *

1) Alcohol Clinical Experimental Research. Mar; 24(3):265-77 - suggested general readings

2) Arbahamson, E.M. (1974) *Body, Mind & Sugar*. New York: Pyramid Books

3) Antoni, M.H.; Cruess, S.; Cruess, D.G.; Kumar, M.; Lutgendorf, S.; Ironson, G.; Dettmer, E.; Williams, J.; Klimas, N.; Fletcher, M.A.; Schneiderman, N. (2000) *Cognitive-behavioral stress management reduces distress and 24-hour urinary free cortisol output among symptomatic HIV-infected gay men*. Annals of Behavioral Medicine. Winter;22(1):29-37.

4) Anthony, Michael & Barbara, Taylor (2008) *Income without a job*. Lulu Publications

5) Avitia, E.; Mendoza-Fernandez, V.; Escobar, A. (2000) *Anxiolytic-like actions of melatonin, 5-metoxytryptophol, 5-hydroxytryptophol and benzodiazepines on a conflict procedure*. Prog Neuropsychopharmacol Biol Psychiatry. Jan; 24(1):117-29.

6) Bandura, Albert (1982) Self-efficacy: *Mechanism in Human Agency*. APA. American Psychologist, Vol. 37, No 2, February

7) Bargh, John (2007) *Social Psychology and the Unconscious: The Automaticity of Higher Mental Processes* Psychology Press: New York

8) Bandyopadhyay, D.; Biswas, K.; Bandyopadhyay, U.; Reiter, R.J.; Banerjee, R.K. (2000) *Melatonin protects against stress-induced gastric lesions by scavenging the hydroxyl radical.* Journal of Pineal Research. Oct; 29(3):143-51.

9) Beck-Friis, J.; Kjellman, B.F.; Aperia, B.; Unden, F.; von Rosen D.; Ljunggren, J.G.; Wetterberg. L. (1985) *Serum melatonin in relation to clinical variables in patientswith major depressive disorder and a hypothesis of a low melatonin syndrome.* Acta Psychiatry Scandinavia. Apr; 71(4):319-30.

10) Bern, R. and M. Levy (1995) *Physiology* Third ed. St. Lousi: Mosby publishing

11) Billett, E.A.; Richter, M.A.; Sam, F.; Swinson, R..; Dai, X.Y.; King, N.; Badri, F.; Sasaki, T.; Buchanan, J.A.; Kennedy, J.L. (1998) *Investigation of dopamine system genes in obsessive-compulsive disorder.* Psychiatry Genetics. Autumn; 8(3):163-9.

12) Biondi, M.; Costantini, A.; Parisi, A. (1996) *Can loss and grief activate latent neoplasia? A clinical case of possible interaction between genetic risks and stress in breast cancer.* Psychotherapy Psychosomatic Mar-Apr; 65(2):102-5.

13) Blankfield, A.; (1983) *Grief and alcohol.* Am J Drug Alcohol Abuse. ; 9(4):435-46.

14) Boyadjieva, N.; Sarkar, D.K. (1999) *Effects of ethanol on basal and adenosine-induced increases in beta-endorphin release and intracellular cAMP levels in hypothalamic cells.* Brain Research. Apr 3; 824(1):112-8.

15) Brennan, Barbara Ann (1993) *Hands of Light.* New York: Bantam Books

16) Buss, David M. (2005) *The Handbook of Evolutionary Psychology.* John Wiley and Sons: Hoboken, NJ

17) Byrne, Rhonda (2006) *The Secret.* Atria Books

18) Cabassi, A.; Bouchard, J.F., Dumont, E.C.; Girouard, H.; Le Jossec, M.; Lamontagne, D.; Besner, J.G.; de Champlain J. (2000) *Effect of antioxidant treatments on nitrate tolerance development in normotensive and hypertensive rats.* Journal of Hypertension. Feb; 18(2):187-96.

19) Calandra, Bob (Mar, 2003). *Be a Stress Buster: Workshops on Dealing with Emotions in the Workplace can Reveal Anxiety-reducing Secrets.* The Scientist. V17 i6 p52 (2)

20) Clayton, P.J. (1990) *Bereavement and depression.* J Clinical Psychiatry. Jul; 51 Suppl: 34-8; discussion 39-40.

21) Cousins, Norman (1985). *Therapeutic Value of Laughter.* Integrative Psychiatry. Vol. 3(2), pp.112

22) Cruess, D.G.; Antoni, M.H.; McGregor, B.A.; Kilbourn, K.M.; Boyers, A.E.; Alferi, S.M.; Carver, C.S.; Kumar, M. (2000*) Cognitive-behavioral stress management reduces serum cortisol by enhancing benefit finding among women being treated for early stage breast cancer.* Psychosomatic Medicine. May-Jun; 62(3):304-8.

23) Dana, Richard H. (1993) *Multicultural Assessment Perspectives for Professional Psychology.* Allyn and Bacon

24) David-Neel, Alexandra (1931) *Initiations and Initiates in Tibet.* Ryder and Company: London

25) De A, Boyadjieva N.I.; Sarkar, D.K. (1990) *Effect of voltage-dependent calcium channel blockers on ethanol-induced beta-endorphin release from hypothalamic neurons in primary cultures*. Alcohol Clinical Experimental Research. May; 23(5):850-5.

26) Deigner, H.P.; Haberkorn, U.; Kinscherf, R. (2000) *Apoptosis modulators in the therapy of neurodegenerative diseases*. Expert Opinion Investigating Drugs. Apr; 9(4):747-64. Review.

27) del Arbol, J.L.; Munoz, J.R.; Ojeda, L.; Cascales, A.L.; Irles, J.R.; Miranda, M.T.; Ruiz, Requena M.E.; Aguirre, J.C. (2000) *Plasma concentrations of beta-endorphin in smokers who consume different numbers of cigarettes per day*. Pharmacology Biochemistry and Behavior.
Sep; 67(1):25-8.

28) Durant, Will (1961) *The Story of Philosophy 2nd Ed.* Simon and Shuster: NY

29) Evans-Wentz, W. Y. (2000) *Tibetan Yoga and the Secret Doctrines*. Oxford University Press

30) Ezekiel, Isaac A. (1966) *Kabir: The great mystic*. Radha Soami Satsang: Beas

31) Folks, D.G. (2004). *The Interface of Psychiatry and Irritable Bowel Syndrome*. Curr Psychiatry Rep. 2004 Jun; 6(3):210-5. E

32) Frazer, Nicole (2002). *Family History of Hypertension is Related to Maladaptive Behavioral Responses as Well as Exaggerated Physiological Reactions to Stress, According to Study.* APA press releases, May 12.

33) Froehlich, J.C.; Zink, R.W.; Li, T.K.; Christian, J.C. (2000) *Analysis of heritability of hormonal responses to alcohol in twins: beta-endorphin as a potential biomarker of genetic risk for alcoholism.* Alcohol Clin Exp Res. 2000 Mar;24(3):265-77

34) Furukawa, T.; Harai, H.; Hirai, T.; Fujihara, S.; Kitamura, T.; Takahashi, K. (1998) *Childhood parental loss and alcohol dependence among Japanese men: a case-control study. Group for Longitudinal Affective Disorders Study (GLADS).* Acta Psychiatry Scandinavia. Jun; 97(6):403-7.

35) Gianoulakis, C. (1996) *Implications of endogenous opioids and dopamine in alcoholism: human and basic science studies*. Alcohol Mar;1:33-42. Review.

36) Glasser, William (1965) *Reality Therapy: A New Approach to Psychiatry.* Perennial Library. Harper and Row

37) Grisel, J.E.; Mogil, J.S.; Grahame, N.J.; Rubinstein, M.; Belknap, J.K., Crabbe, J.C.; Low, M.J. (1999) *Ethanol oral self-administration is increased in mutant mice with decreased beta-endorphin expression.* Brain Research. Jul 17; 835(1):62-7.

38) Haeri Shaykh Fadialla (1990) *The Elements of Sufism.* Elements Books Limited

39) Hall, M.; Buysse, D.J.; Dew, M.A.; Prigerson, H.G.; Kupfer, D.J.; Reynolds, C.F. (1997) *Intrusive thoughts and avoidance behaviors are associated with sleep disturbances in bereavement-related depression.* Depression and Anxiety. 6(3):106-12.

40) Hall, Manly, P. (1978) *The Secret Teachings of All Ages: An Encyclopedic Outline of Masonic, Hermetic, Qabbalistic & Rosicrucian Symbolical. Philosophy.* Philosophical Research Society Inc.

41) Heeg, Theresa (Oct, 2003). *Don't Let Stress Make Your Workplace Unhealthy.* Aspen Publishers: Patient care management. v19i10p5 (2)

42) Hofer, M.A. (1996) *On the nature and consequences of early loss.* Psychosomatic Medicine. Nov-Dec; 58(6):570-81.

43) Horakova, L.; Ondrejickova, O.; Bachrata K.; Vajdova. M. (2000*) Preventive effect of several antioxidants after oxidative stress on rat brain homogenates.* General Physiological Biophysics. Jun; 19(2):195-205.

44) Hubbard, L. Ron (2007) *Dianetics: The modern science of mental health.* Bridge Publication Inc..

45) Hubbard, L. Ron (1975) *Dianetics Today* Church of Scientology of California Publications

46) Hubbard, L. Ron (1951) *Science of Survival: Prediction of Human Behavior*, Bridge Publications: Los Angeles, CA

47) Hubbard, L. Ron (1952) *Scientology: A History of Man.* Bridge Publications: Los Angeles, CA

48) Hubbard, L. Ron (1955) *The Creation of Human Ability.* Bridge Publications: Los Angeles, CA

49) Hunter, R.J. (2005). *Pastoral Counseling.* Dictionary of Pastoral Care and Counseling. Nashville: Abingdon Press.

50) Jacobs, S.C.; Mason, J.W.; Kosten, T.R.; Wahby V.; Kasl S.V.; Ostfeld, A.M. (1986) *Bereavement and catecholamines*. J Psychosomatic Research. 30(4):489-96.

51) Johnson, Julian (1985) *The Path of the Masters* 14th ed. Radha Soami Sat Sang: Beas

52) Juszczak, M.; Bojanowska, E.; Guzek, J.W.; Stempniak, B.; Dabrowski, R. (1999)*The effect of melatonin on vasopressin release under stress conditions in pinealectomized male rats.* Adv Exp Med Biol.; 460:311-5.

53) Kajdaniuk, D.; Marek, B.; Swietochowska, E.; Ciesielska-Kopacz, N.; Buntner, B. (2000) *Is positive correlation between cortisol and met-enkephalin concentration in blood of women with breast cancer a reaction to stress before chemotherapy administration?* Pathophysiology. Apr; 7(1):47-51.

54) Kato, K.; Asai, S.; Murai, I.; Nagata, T.; Takahashi, Y.; Komuro, S.; Iwasaki, A.; Ishikawa, K.; Arakawa, Y. (2001) *Melatonin's gastroprotective and antistress roles involve both central and peripheral effects.* Journal of Gastroenterology. Feb; 36(2):91-5.

55) Katz, V.L.; Warren, M.; Ekstrom, R.D.; Mason, G.; Heine, A.; Golden, R. (1999) *Psychobiological markers of stress in pregnancy: 6-sulfatoxymelatonin—a longitudinal study.* American J Perinatology. 16(5):233-8.

56) Keil, Frank. (1998) *Developmental Psychology.* In press

57) King, Godfre Ray (1934) *Unveiled Mysteries*. Saint Germain Press.

58) King, Godfre Ray (1934) *The Magic Presence*. Saint Germain Press

59) Kirby, A.W.; Clayton, M.; Rivera, P.; Comperatore, C.A. (1999) *Melatonin and the reduction or alleviation of stress*. J Pineal Research. Sep; 27(2):78-85.

60) Khan, Hazrat Inayat (1983) *The Music of Life*. Omega Press: Santa Fe, NM

61) Klemp, Harold (2004) *The Art of Spiritual Dreaming*. Eckankar: Minneapolis, MN

62) Klemp, Harold (1997) *The Spiritual Exercises of Eck*. Echankar: Minneapolis, MN

64) Klimas, N.; Fletcher, M.A.; Schneiderman, N. (2000) *Cognitive-behavioral stress management reduces distress and 24-hour urinary free cortisol output among symptomatic HIV-infected gay men*. Annals of Behavioral Medicine. Winter;22(1):29-37.

65) Kopp, C.; Vogel, E.; Rettori, M.C.; Delagrange, P.; Misslin, R. (1999) *The effects of melatonin on the behavioral disturbances induced by chronic mild stress in C3H/He mice*. Behavioral Pharmacology. Feb; 10(1):73-83.

66) Kosten, T.R.; Jacobs, S.; Mason, J.W. (1984) *The dexamethasone suppression test during bereavement.* J Nervous Mental Disorders. Jun; 172(6):359-60.

67) Kravetz, Robert E. (2008) *Medical Humanism: Aphorisms from the bedside teachings & writings of Howard M. Spiro, MD.* Buse Printing

68) Linnard-Palmer, L. and S. Kools (Jan, 2005) *Parents' refusal of medical treatment for cultural or religious beliefs: an ethnographic study of health care professionals' experiences.* J Pediatr Oncol Nurs. 2005 Jan-Feb; 22(1):48-57.

69) Maestroni, G.J. (2001) *The immunotherapeutic potential of melatonin.* Expert Opinion Investigating Drugs. Mar; 10(3):467-76.

70) Maltz, Maxwell (1960) *Psycho-Cybernetics: A New Way to Get More Living out of Life.* Prentice Hall

71) Martikainen, P. and T. Valkonen (1996) *Mortality after the death of a spouse: rates and causes of death in a large Finnish cohort.* American J Public Health. Aug; 86(8 Pt 1):1087-93.

72) Maslov, L.N.; Krylatov, A.V.; Lishmanov, I.B. (1999) *The anti-arrhythmic activity of agonists of the peripheral mu-opiate Receptors.* Eksp Klin Farmakol. May-Jun; 62(3):28-31.

73) McGrady, A.; Bailey, B.K.; Good, M.P. (1991)

Controlled study of biofeedback-assisted relaxation in type I diabetes. Diabetes Care. May;14(5):360-5.

74) Medlin, Douglas L.; Ross, Brian H.; Arthur Markman (2005) *Cognitive Psychology 4th Ed.* John Wiley and Sons: Hoboken, NJ

75) Mellstrom, D.; Nilsson, A.; Oden, A.; Rundgren, A.; Svanborg, A. (1982) *Mortality among the widowed in Sweden.* Scand J Social Medicine. 10(2):33-41.

76) Morioka, N.; Okatani, Y.; Wakatsuki, A. (1999) *Melatonin protects against age-related DNA damage in the brains of female senescence-accelerated mice.* Journal of Pineal Research. Nov; 27(4):202-9.

77) Moss, R. (2000) *Cardiology Essentials.* Independent study course manual. Madison: University of Wisconsin-Madison School of Medicine.

78) Naranjo-Rodriguez, E.B.; Osornio, A.O.; Hernandez-Reiter, R.J.; Tan, D.X.; Osuna. C.; Gitto, E. (2000) *Actions of melatonin in the reduction of oxidative stress.* A review. Journal of Biomedical Science. Nov-Dec; 7(6):444-58. Review

79) Nolen-Hoeksema, Susan (2008) *Abnormal Psychology 4th ed.* McGraw-Hill: NY

80) O'Connor, Joe. *God and the Brain. Is Belief a Psychological Condition? A collection of great articles on the subject.*
http://atheistempire.com/reference/brain/main.html

81) Okatani, Y.; Wakatsuki, A.; Reiter, R.J. (2000) *Protective effect of melatonin against homocysteine-induced vasoconstriction of human umbilical artery.* Biochemical Biophysics Res Commun. Oct 22; 277(2):470-5.

82) Pasero, Christine (1998) *Pain Control: Is Laughter the best Medicine?* The American Journal of Nursing. Vol. 98, No 12, Dec, pp. 12+14

83) Pfeiffer, C. (1975) *Mental and Elemental Elements.* New Canaan, CT: Keats Publishing

84) Powell, A. E. (1928) *The Causal Body.* The Theosophical Publishing House: London

85) Prigerson, H.G. (2001) *Grief and its relation to posttraumatic stress disorder.* Post Traumatic Stress Disorder: Diagnosis, Management and Treatment: Martin Dunitz Publisher

86) Quinlan, Jay. *Psychoneuroimmunology.*
http://www.nfnlp.com/psychoneuroimmunology_quinlan.htm#intro

87) Rosenbaum, L. (1983) *Biofeedback-assisted stress*

management for insulin-treated diabetes mellitus. <u>Biofeedback and Self Regulation</u>. Dec; 8(4):519-32.

88) Rosenthal, N. & M. Blehar (1989*). Seasonal affective disorders and phototherapy.* New York: Guilford Press

89) Ruzich, M.; Martin-Iverson, M.T. (2000) *Pinealectomy blocks stress-induced motor stimulation but not sensitization and tolerance to a dopamine D2 receptor agonist.* <u>Psychopharmacology (Berl)</u>. Oct; 152(3):275-82.

90) Ryushi, T. et al (1998). *The Effect of Exposure to Negative Air Ions on the Recovery of Physiological Responses after Moderate Endurance Exercise.* Int J Biometeorol. 1998 Feb; 41(3):132-6.

91) Safety Compliance Letter. (Aug, 2003). *Creating a Safe and Stress-free Workplace.* Aspen Publishers. i2431 p5 (2)

92) Schacter, Daniel, L.; Gilbert, Daniel T.; and Daniel M. Wegner. *Psychology.* Worth Publishers

93) Schleifer, S.J.; Keller, S.E.; Camerino, M.; Thornton, J.C.; Stein, M. (1983) *Supression of lymphocyte stimulation following bereavement.* JAMA. Jul 15; 250(3):374-7.

94) Shamir, E.; Rotenberg, V.S.; Laudon, M.; Zisapel, N.; Elizur, A. (2000) *First-night effect of melatonin treatment in patients with chronic schizophrenia.* Journal of Clinical Psychopharmacology. Dec; 20(6):691-4.

95) Shepherd, Gordon M. (1990) *The Synaptic Organization of the Brain 3rd ed.* Oxford University Press

96) Shuchter, S.R.; Zisook, S.; Kirkorowicz, C.; Risch C. (1986*) The dexamethasone suppression test in acute grief.* American J Psychiatry. Jul; 143(7):879-81.

97) Sibarov, D.A.; Kovalenko, R.I.; Nozdrachev, A.D. (2000) *Pinealocyte functioning in stress during daytime in rats. Ross Fiziol Zh Im I M Sechenova.* Aug; 86(8):1049-56.

98) Singh, Kirpal (1981) *The Jap Ji: The Message of Guru Nanak.* Sawan Kirpal Publications

99) Singh, Shiv Dayal (2002) *Sar Bachan Poetry.* Beas: Radha Soami Sat Sang

100) Singh Shiv Dayal (1991) *Sar Bachan Prose 9th Ed.* Beas: Radha Saomi Sat Sang

101) Skaper, S.D.; Floreani., M.; Ceccon, M.; Facci, L.; Giusti, P. (1999) *Excitotoxicity, oxidative stress,*

and the neuroprotective potential of melatonin. Ann N Y Acad Sci. 890:107-18. Review

102) Sturman, G. (1996) *Histaminergic drugs as modulators of CNS function.* Pflugers Archives. 431(6 Suppl 2):R223-4.

103) Syvalahti, E.; Eskola, J.; Ruuskanen, O.; Laine, T. (1985) *Nonsuppression of cortisol in depression and immune function.* Prog Neuropsychopharmacol Biol Psychiatry. 9(4):413-22.

104) Thurman, Robert (trans.) (1994) *The Tibetan Book of the Dead, as popularly known in the West; known in Tibet as "The Great Book of Natural)Liberation Through Understanding in the Between.* London: Harper Collins

105) Twitchell, Paul. (1969) *Eckankar the Key to Secret Worlds.* Illuminated Way Press

106) Twitchell, Paul. (1971) *The Spiritual Notebook.* Illuminated Way Press

107) Volpicelli, J.; Balaraman, G.; Hahn, J.; Wallace H.; Bux, D. (1999) *The role of uncontrollable trauma in the development of PTSD and alcohol addiction.* Alcohol Res Health. 23(4):256-62.

108) Wakatsuki, A; Okatani, Y.; Shinohara, K.; Ikenoue, N.; Kaneda, C.; Fukaya, T. (2001) *Melatonin protects fetal rat brain against oxidative mitochondrial damage*. Journal Pineal Research. Jan; 30(1):22-8.

109) Weller, E.B.; Weller, R.A.; Fristad, M.A.; Bowes, J.M. (1990) *Dexamethasone suppression test and depressive symptoms in bereaved children: a preliminary report*. J Neuropsychiatry Clin Neurosci. Fall; 2(4):418-21.

110) Wikipedia: *Subatomic particles*
http://en.wikipedia.org/wiki/Subatomic_particleW

111) Wikipedia: *Galaxies* -
http://en.wikipedia.org/wiki/Galaxy

112) *Wikipedia:* Multiverse -
http://en.wikipedia.org/wiki/Multiverse

113) Wilkins, Julia and Amy J. Eisenbraum (2009). *Humor Theories and the Physiological Benefits of Laughter*. Holistic Nursing Practice. Vol 23, Issue 6, p 349-354

114) Wurtman, R. & J. Weisel (1969) *Environmental lighting and neuroendrocrine function. Relationships between spectrum of light source and gonadal growth.*

Endocrinology, 85: 1218

115) Van Gelder, Dora (1977) *The Real World of Faires*. The Theosophical Publishing House

116) Yogananda, Paramhansa (2005) *Autobiography of a Yogi*. Crystal Clarity Publishers

117) Yogi, Maharishi, Mahesh (1963) *The Science of Being and the Art of Living: Transcendental Meditation*. Penguin Books: New York

118) Zelena, D.; Kiem, D.T.; Barna, I.; Makara, G.B. (1999) *Alpha 2-adrenoreceptor subtypes regulate ACTH and beta-endorphin secretions during stress in the rat*. Psychoneuroendocrinology. Apr;24(3):333-43.

119) Basso. Jr., M.R. (2001) *Neurobiological Relationships Between Ambient Lighting and the Startle Response to Acoustic Stress in Humans*. International Journal of Neuroscience vol. 10

120 Lieber, Deborah (1986) *Laughter and Humor in Critical Care*. Dimensions of Critical Care Nursing. May/June Vol 5 Issue 3

121 Hollwich, F. and B. Dieckhues (1980) *The effect of natural and artificial light via the eye on the hormonal and metabolic balance of animals and man*. Opthalmologia, 180, (4), 188-97

122 Osaka, Y. and R. Wurtman (1978) *Spectral power distribution of light sources affects growth and development f rats.* Photochemistry and Photobiology, vol 29, Great Britain: Pergamon Press

123 Ott, J. (1974) *The eyes dual function part I.* Eye Ear Nose and Throat Monthly, Vol 53

124 Wurtman, R. (1975) *The effects of light on man and other mammals.* Lab report: Department of Nutrition and Food Science. Cambridge: MIT Press

125 Leibermann, J. (1991) *Light: Medicine of the Future.* Santa Fe: Bear and Company

*Please note that this abbreviated list of references and suggested readings is just a brief overview of relevant topics pertaining to *Spiritual Medicine* and that they are included for information only.

These materials do not necessarily represent the views, opinions, ethical positions or vested interests of the author.

The list includes materials that may seem controversial to some readers. That's Ok, and in fact the uncomfortable materials are often the ones that you may learn the most from.

Authority without truth is meaningless; while truth without authority is the much wiser choice.

Lux et Sonas et Veritas *

*Light and Sound and Truth

Insights:

Insights:

www.ingramcontent.com/pod-product-compliance
Lightning Source LLC
Chambersburg PA
CBHW031835170526
45157CB00001B/305